IFMBE Proceedings

Volume 81

The IFMBE Proceedings Book Series is an official publication of *the International Federation for Medical and Biological Engineering* (IFMBE). The series gathers the proceedings of various international conferences, which are either organized or endorsed by the Federation. Books published in this series report on cutting-edge findings and provide an informative survey on the most challenging topics and advances in the fields of medicine, biology, clinical engineering, and biophysics.

The series aims at disseminating high quality scientific information, encouraging both basic and applied research, and promoting world-wide collaboration between researchers and practitioners in the field of Medical and Biological Engineering.

Topics include, but are not limited to:

- Diagnostic Imaging, Image Processing, Biomedical Signal Processing
- Modeling and Simulation, Biomechanics
- Biomaterials, Cellular and Tissue Engineering
- Information and Communication in Medicine, Telemedicine and e-Health
- Instrumentation and Clinical Engineering
- Surgery, Minimal Invasive Interventions, Endoscopy and Image Guided Therapy
- Audiology, Ophthalmology, Emergency and Dental Medicine Applications
- Radiology, Radiation Oncology and Biological Effects of Radiation

IFMBE proceedings are indexed by by SCOPUS, EI Compendex, Japanese Science and Technology Agency (JST), SCImago.

Proposals can be submitted by contacting the Springer responsible editor shown on the series webpage (see "Contacts"), or by getting in touch with the series editor Ratko Magjarevic.

More information about this series at http://www.springer.com/series/7403

Fatimah Ibrahim · Juliana Usman ·
Mohd Yazed Ahmad · Norhamizan Hamzah
Editors

3rd International Conference for Innovation in Biomedical Engineering and Life Sciences

Proceedings of ICIBEL 2019,
December 6–7, 2019, Kuala Lumpur, Malaysia

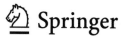 Springer

Editors
Fatimah Ibrahim
Department of Biomedical Engineering
University of Malaya
Kuala Lumpur, Malaysia

Juliana Usman
Department of Biomedical Engineering
University of Malaya
Kuala Lumpur, Malaysia

Mohd Yazed Ahmad
Department of Biomedical Engineering
University of Malaya
Kuala Lumpur, Malaysia

Norhamizan Hamzah
Department of Rehabilitation Medicine
University of Malaya
Kuala Lumpur, Kuala Lumpur, Malaysia

ISSN 1680-0737   ISSN 1433-9277   (electronic)
IFMBE Proceedings
ISBN 978-3-030-65091-9   ISBN 978-3-030-65092-6   (eBook)
https://doi.org/10.1007/978-3-030-65092-6

This Springer imprint is published by the registered company Springer Nature Switzerland AG
The registered company address is: Gewerbestrasse 11, 6330 Cham, Switzerland

Preface

Development of medical devices requires an exchange of thought and ideas between engineers and medical researchers, and this can be difficult in light of the very different technical languages spoken by these two groups. The 2019 International Conference in Biomedical Engineering and Life sciences held in Kuala Lumpur, from December 6–7, 2019, offered a unique platform to facilitate this necessary exchange.

This volume includes 19 peer-reviewed papers relating to timely issues in biomechanics, ergonomics and rehabilitation, biosensing and life sciences, as well as solutions for technology transfer, telemedicine and point of care healthcare. The main review criteria were: the relevance to the conference, the contribution to academic debate, the appropriateness of the research method and the clarity of the presented result. The acceptance rate was 63%.

This biannual conference will not have been possible without the endless dedication of the conference committee, the Center of Innovation in Medical Engineering (CIME) University of Malaya, UM Center of Innovation and Commercialization (UMCIC), the Faculty of Engineering UM, MSMBE, IFMBE, sponsors, reviewers, speakers, presenters and delegates. We would like to thank all of them and hope that this book can offer a faithful record of the topics discussed at the event and a source of inspiration for new ideas and collaboration.

Fatimah Ibrahim
Juliana Usman
Mohd Yazed Ahmad
Norhamizan Hamzah

Conference Details

Name

3rd International Conference for Innovation in Biomedical Engineering and Life Sciences
In conjunction with
1st World Congress on Falls and Postural Stability 2019

Short Name

ICIBEL2019 and WCFPS2019

Venue

6th December 2019
Kuala Lumpur Convention Center (KLCC), Kuala Lumpur, Malaysia

7th December 2019
Pullman KLCC, Kuala Lumpur, Malaysia

Proceedings Editors

Fatimah Ibrahim
Juliana Usman
Mohd Yazed Bin Ahmad
Norhamizan Hamzah

Organized by

University of Malaya, Malaysia
Center for Innovation in Medical Engineering (CIME)

Co-organized by

Malaysia's Society of Medical and Biological Engineering (MSMBE)

Endorsed by

International Federation for Medical and Biological Engineering (IFMBE)

Supported by

IFMBE Asia Pacific Working Group
IEEE University of Malaya Student Branch
University of Malaya Centre of Innovation & Commercialization (UMCIC)
Medical Device Authority (MDA), Ministry of Health Malaysia
Tourism Malaysia

Organizing Committee

Chairperson

Fatimah Ibrahim   Faculty of Engineering, University of Malaya,
                              Malaysia

Co-chair

Tan Maw Pin   Faculty of Medicine, University of Malaya,
                              Malaysia

Publication

Fatimah Ibrahim   Faculty of Engineering, University of Malaya,
                              Malaysia
Juliana Usman   Faculty of Engineering, University of Malaya,
                              Malaysia

Secretary

Noraisyah Mohamed Shah   Faculty of Engineering, University of Malaya,
                              Malaysia

Treasurer

Mas Sahidayana Mohktar   Faculty of Engineering, University of Malaya,
                              Malaysia

Publicity/Logistic

Norhayati Soin   Faculty of Engineering, University of Malaya,
                              Malaysia

Technical

Mohd Yazed Ahmad	Faculty of Engineering, University of Malaya, Malaysia
Wan Safwani Wan Kamarul Zaman	Faculty of Engineering, University of Malaya, Malaysia
Norhamizan Hamzah	Faculty of Medicine, University of Malaya, Malaysia
Teh Swe Jyan	Faculty of Engineering, University of Malaya, Malaysia
Chan Chow Khuen	Faculty of Engineering, University of Malaya, Malaysia
Lee Ching Shya	UMCIC, University of Malaya, Malaysia
Siti Munirah Md Noh	UMCIC, University of Malaya, Malaysia

Sponsorship/Exhibition

Wan Safwani Wan Kamarul Zaman	Faculty of Engineering, University of Malaya, Malaysia

Secretariat Committee

Wan Safwani Wan Kamarul Zaman	Faculty of Engineering, University of Malaya, Malaysia
Mohd Faiz Zulkeflee	Faculty of Engineering, University of Malaya, Malaysia
Yuslialif Mohd Yusup	Faculty of Engineering, University of Malaya, Malaysia
Izaidah Jamaludin	UMCIC, University of Malaya, Malaysia
Siti Nurul 'Ashikin Sabaruddin	UMCIC, University of Malaya, Malaysia

International Advisory Board

Yu Haoyong	National University Singapore, Singapore
Marc J. Madou	University California, Irvine, USA
Shankar Krishna	International Federation for Medical and Biological Engineering, (IFMBE), USA
Salvador Borros	Universidad Ramon Llull, Spain
Elman El Bakri	Society of Medical and Biological Engineering Malaysia (MSMBE), Malaysia
Azman Hamid	Society of Medical and Biological Engineering Malaysia (MSMBE), Malaysia
Chandra S. Sharma	Indian Institute of Technology, Hyderabad, India
Tei-fu Li	Tsinghua University, China
Sasikala Devi Thangavelu	Medical Device Authority, Ministry of Health, Malaysia
Samsilah Roslan	University Putra Malaysia, Malaysia

Contents

Theme: Medical Devices and Clinical Healthcare

Parameter Identification and Identifiability Analysis for Patient-Induced Effort in Respiratory Mechanics Models

Johnston Lee Teong Jeen[(⊠)], Chiew Yeong Shiong,
and Ganesaramachandran Arunachalam

School of Engineering, Monash University, Selangor, Malaysia
johnstonlee96@gmail.com,
{Chiew.Yeong.Shiong,Ganesaramachandran.Arunachalam}@monash.edu

Abstract. A growing concern in the field of mechanical ventilation (MV) treatment is the lack of optimal patient-specific ventilator setting and automation for spontaneously breathing patients. Model-based respiratory mechanics have been introduced as a non-invasive method of performing respiratory mechanics estimation. In volume-control ventilation (VC), patient's spontaneous effort causes anomalies in the airway pressure reading, which cause alterations in the airway pressure delivered. As a result, MV patient's respiratory mechanics cannot be determined for treatment purposes. To remedy this, a '*polynomial model*' was investigated and the results show a practically nonidentifiable model. In this study, a '*sine-wave model*' where a sinusoidal function added to the single compartment model to describe and capture the patient effort is presented. Monte-Carlo Analysis and identifiability analysis was carried out to determine the performance and stability of the sine-wave model. The results of this study indicate that the sine-wave model fits pressure waveforms with patient effort well but it is practically nonidentifiable in some cases. Misidentification of respiratory mechanics arises when critical characteristics of the pressure waveform are unexpressed. Future research should be focused on models that are not extensions of the single compartment model.

Keywords: Mechanical ventilation · Parameter identification · Identifiability analysis · Respiratory mechanics models

1 Introduction

The field of respiratory mechanics has experienced significant development in recent years due to technological advancements, which has enabled researchers to introduce new ideas, exchange information and communicate effectively. As such, model-based estimation of respiratory mechanics has garnered increasing attention as a method of identifying the mechanical properties of the respiratory system from patient-to-patient, non-invasively [1, 2]. The mechanics of a respiratory system is generally described by the elastance (E) and resistance (R) which is the ability to return to its initial volume

© Springer Nature Switzerland AG 2021
F. Ibrahim et al. (Eds.): ICIBEL 2019, IFMBE Proceedings 81, pp. 3–13, 2021.
https://doi.org/10.1007/978-3-030-65092-6_1

after stretching and to oppose the inflow of air [3]. This information will allow clinicians to (i) diagnose patients for respiratory disease; (ii) monitor the patient condition; (iii) improve patient-ventilator interaction which will inherently minimize the risk of ventilator-induced lung injuries (VILI) [3, 5].

Accurate estimation of patient-specific respiratory mechanics proves to be a challenge for a spontaneously breathing patient whilst on ventilator support, which significantly alters breathing waveforms in an unpredictable manner [1, 6]. Akoumianaki et al. [7] describes a phenomenon named 'ventilator-induced reverse-triggering' whereby patient effort during ventilator support disguises the true, unaffected respiratory system mechanics. In volume-control (VC) mode, this spontaneous patient effort is reflected as a drop in the airway pressure data [6]. Despite its accuracy for passive patients, the widely used single compartment model least square method does not perform well for spontaneously breathing patients. This is because the pressure (due to the respiratory muscles) (P_{mus}) is no longer negligible [3, 6]. Patient inspiratory effort reduces the net airway pressure for a given volume (and flow), which results in a lower calculated elastance [8, 9]. Therefore, respiratory models that are invulnerable to a parameter trade-off is needed to capture the respiratory mechanics of spontaneously breathing patients [9].

To overcome the limitation of the *single compartment model* for spontaneous breaths, Redmond et al. [6] presents a polynomial model of patient breathing effort. This model assumes that the patient effort to be a polynomial function (P_e) in addition to the *single compartment model*. Equation (1) shows this polynomial patient effort function.

$$P_e(t) = \begin{cases} 0, & t < t_s \\ at^2 + bt + c, & t_s \leq t < t_f \\ 0, & t \geq t_f \end{cases} \tag{1}$$

Compared to the conventional *single compartment model*, the polynomial model has less fitting error and more stable estimates of E and R [6]. However, the polynomial model does yield erratic parameter identification for patient efforts that occur early and for long durations, as observed from the large confidence intervals in the identified parameters [6].

Chee et al. [2] builds upon the polynomial model introduced by Redmond et al. [6] by introducing a 'one-second pause' at the end-of-inspiration. The addition of inspiration pause improves the consistency and accuracy of identifying respiratory mechanics parameters [2]. However, the pause is an additional procedure to the ventilation treatment and limits the patient's airflow, rendering it unsuitable for clinical applications. Additionally, the identifiability of model parameters was determined following the method described by Raue et al. [10]. They examined the profile likelihood (SSE) to determine if the model is structurally and practically identifiable and found it to be practically nonidentifiable due to erratic patient efforts [2].

Vicario et al. [3] presents a non-invasive method suitable for real-time patient monitoring using only measurements of airway pressure and flow which is accessible for patients undergoing MV treatment. The method uses a cost function for a constrained optimization approach derived from the *single compartment model* which includes a patient effort function (P_{mus}) as a sinusoidal function [3]. The cost function is written as

$$J = \sum_{k=1}^{k=N} \left(P_{aw}(t_k) - \left(R\dot{V}(t_k) + EV(t_k) + P_{mus}(t_k)\right)\right)^2 \qquad (2)$$

subjected to the physiological constraints of E_{max} and R_{max} which are always positive and P_{mus} is defined as

$$P_{mus}(t) = \begin{cases} P_{str}\sin\left(\frac{\pi}{2t_p}t\right) for\ 0 \le t < t_p \\ P_{str}\sin\left(\frac{\pi}{2(t_r-t_p)}(t+t_r-2t_p)\right) for\ t_p \le t < t_r \\ 0 \quad for\ t_r \le t < t_N \end{cases} \qquad (3)$$

Both simulation and real animal data results show accurate and consistent real-time estimation of the respiratory mechanics, which is suitable for diagnosis and therapy optimization [3]. The results prove that the model is able to continuously estimate the respiratory elastance and resistance for both passively and actively breathing patients undergoing ventilator treatment [3]. The main limitation of this method is that it assumes patient effort always occur at the start of inspiration. Therefore, this method is not suitable for patient-induced breaths that occur at other times.

Combining the previously described studies, the current study will investigate the performance of a model with a modified patient effort sinusoidal function (P_{mus}) to overcome the limitations of the polynomial model [6]. Figure 1 shows the improved model performance of the sine wave model over the single compartment model for

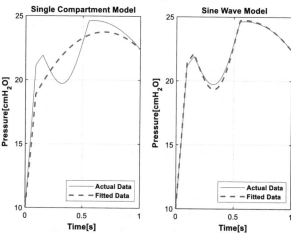

Fig. 1. Model fitting of pressure data with patient effort using a single compartment model and a sine wave model. (*Left*) The single compartment model does not capture the effect of patient effort resulting in poor respiratory mechanics estimation. (*Right*) The sine wave model can capture the effect of patient effort to enable accurate respiratory mechanics estimation.

spontaneously breathing waveforms. The analysis procedure for respiratory mechanics models will be adopted from Chee et al. [2]. Generally, the results from this study seeks to contribute further investigation into effective MV treatment for actively breathing patients experiencing respiratory failure such as acute respiratory distress syndrome (ARDS) [11].

2 Methodology

2.1 The Sine-Wave Model

The widely accepted single compartment linear lung model as defined in [13] is written as:

$$P_{aw}(t) = E_{lung}V(t) + R_{lung}\dot{V}(t) + P_o \tag{4}$$

where P_{aw} is airway pressure (cmH$_2$O), E is the patient-specific lung elastance (cmH$_2$O/L), V is the inspiratory volume (L), R is the patient-specific lung resistance (cmH$_2$O•s/L), $\dot{V}$ is the inspiratory flow (L/s), t is time (s), and P_o is the offset pressure or PEEP (cmH$_2$O) [14]. Based on the suggestion by Redmond et al. [6], a sine function which represents patient respiratory muscle effort [3] is modified from Eq. (3) and added to the single compartment model to become:

$$P_{aw}(t) = E_{lung}V(t) + R_{lung}\dot{V}(t) + P_o + P_e(t) \tag{5}$$

where by P_e is the patient effort function and is defined as:

$$P_e(t) = \begin{cases} 0 & for\ t \leq t_s \\ P_{str}sin\left(\frac{\pi}{2(t_p - t_s)}(2t_p - t - t_s)\right) & for\ t_s < t \leq t_p \\ P_{str}sin\left(\frac{\pi}{2(t_f - t_p)}(t + t_f - 2t_p)\right) & for\ t_p < t \leq t_f \\ 0\ for\ t > t_f \end{cases} \tag{6}$$

where by the function dictates zero patient effort for time ranges of ($t \leq t_s$) and ($t > t_f$). Equation (6) separates the patient effort function into two portions, decreasing and increasing concave sine functions of the same P_{str} for time ranges.
  ($t_s < t \leq t_p$) and ($t_p < t \leq t_f$) respectively (see Fig. 2).

2.2 Forward Simulation and Parameter Identification

Forward simulation was adopted instead of actual patient data in order for controlled analysis of model performance, for different parameter combinations. Simulations were performed using MATLAB (2018b, MathWorks, Natick, MA). In volume-control ventilation (VCV), flow ($\dot{V}$) can be delivered in several predetermined flow profiles such as constant, ramped, or sinusoidal [15]. For comparison with the polynomial model in previous literature [2, 6], a ramp flow profile was used. Likewise, inspiration is assumed to occur within one second. A ramp flow profile delivers flowrate rapidly at the start of inspiration from 0 until 1, followed by a gradual decrease in flow back to zero.

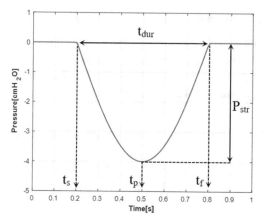

Fig. 2. Representation of time values for the sine wave model. Where t_s is the start time of patient effort, t_f is the end time of patient effort, t_{dur} is the duration of patient effort, P_{str} is the strength of patient effort and t_p is the time at which P_{str} is maximum.

From the simulated flow data, volume (V) is calculated by integrating flow ($\dot{V}$) [11]. To find P_{aw}, which is the forward simulated airway pressure, Eq. (5) was solved using Eq. (6) and parameter values as shown in Table 1. Next, 1000 samples of 10% random normally distributed noise which replicated the perturbations found in actual patient data were added. From the noisy pressure data, set respiratory mechanics parameters, and specified patient effort time, a parameter identification method [12] was used to determine respiratory mechanics. To remain consistent with the previous study [2], Multiple Linear Regression (MLR) was adopted as the parameter identification method. For this, Eq. (5) is rewritten as a matrix to utilize the MATLAB backslash (\) function.

$$
\begin{bmatrix}
V(t_o) & \dot{V}(t_o) & 0 \\
\vdots & \vdots & \vdots \\
V(t_s) & \dot{V}(t_s) & \sin(\ldots t_s) \\
\vdots & \vdots & \vdots \\
V(t_p) & \dot{V}(t_p) & \sin(\ldots t_p) \\
\vdots & \vdots & \vdots \\
V(t_f) & \dot{V}(t_f) & \sin(\ldots t_f) \\
\vdots & \vdots & \vdots \\
V(t) & \dot{V}(t) & \sin(\ldots t)
\end{bmatrix}
\times
\begin{bmatrix}
E \\
R \\
P_{str}
\end{bmatrix}
=
\begin{bmatrix}
P(t_o) - PEEP \\
\vdots \\
P(t_s) - PEEP \\
\vdots \\
P(t_p) - PEEP \\
\vdots \\
P(t_f) - PEEP \\
\vdots \\
P(t) - PEEP
\end{bmatrix}
\tag{7}
$$

2.3 Stability and Performance of Sine-Wave Model

To examine the model stability for a variety of breaths, Monte-Carlo analysis was carried out in this simulation [16]. All model parameters were varied as shown in Table 1 except PEEP which was fixed at a value of 10 cmH$_2$O. Extensive research has been documented by Chiew et al. [13] on the optimization of PEEP during MV treatment.

Table 1. Range of Parameters used for Monte-Carlo Analysis

Parameter	Parameter range	Step size
E	[20]–[36]	2
R	[5]–[15]	2
t_s	[−1]–[1]	0.1
t_{dur}	[0]–[1.2]	0.1
P_{str}	[−4]–[-16]	2

Various combinations of Elastance (E) and Resistance (R) produces different airway pressure waveforms. Parameters t_s, t_{dur} and P_{str} affect the start, duration and amplitude of patient effort respectively in the breath cycle. Patient-induced effort can occur anytime during MV treatment. This includes before the start of ventilator supported breath where $t < 0$ s. In addition, the duration of the breath can be very short or longer than the ventilator inspiration time ($t > 1$ s). Including the 1000 noise samples of each breath, the Monte-Carlo analysis for the sine wave model is conducted for 103,194,000 unique breath cycles.

The Absolute Percentage Error (APE) between the identified parameters and predetermined parameters were calculated. APE is the percentage difference of the identified parameter from its true value which reflects on the performance of the sine wave model.

$$APE(\%) = \left| \frac{E_{Identified} - E_{actual}}{E_{actual}} \right| \times 100 \qquad (8)$$

2.4 Identifiability Analysis of the Sine-Wave Model

From the identified parameters upon solving Eq. (7), these values are input into Eq. (5) to re-simulate the airway pressure. The re-simulated airway pressure is a fitting of the actual airway pressure with patient effort using the sine-wave model. To investigate the quality of model fitting [2, 10, 17], the Sum of Square Error (SSE) is calculated as shown in Eq. (9). The SSE contours were also plotted to analyze the identifiability of model parameters.

$$SSE = |P_{resim} - P_{actual}|^2 \qquad (9)$$

3 Results

From the simulations, samples of patient effort conditions were identified for further analysis. Figure 3 shows four examples of successful parameter identification each with a different case of patient effort observed from the Monte-Carlo Analysis. Conversely, Fig. 4 shows four examples of unsuccessful parameter identification with different cases of patient effort observed from the Monte-Carlo Analysis. Also, Table 2 and Table 3 shows the median and interquartile range of identified parameters E, R and Pstr for the successful and unsuccessful parameter identification cases respectively.

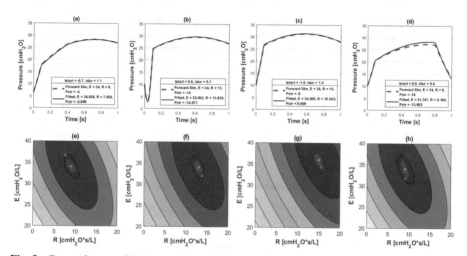

Fig. 3. Cases of successful sine-wave model fitting and parameter identification for breaths with patient effort. (*Top Row*) Plot of forward simulated pressure curve and the fitted sine-wave model. (*Bottom Row*) SSE contours for identifiability analysis of the respective cases above it. (Red Cross: Pairs of E and R from MLR parameter identification, Cyan Asterisk: Center of cluster, and Green Circle: Worst parameter identified pair used to plot fitted curve).

4 Discussion

4.1 Comparison with the Polynomial Model

The performance of the sine-wave model is compared to the polynomial model [2, 6] for actively and passively breathing patients. From the results, it is evident that the sine-wave model has better model fitting and stability. From Table 2 and Table 3, the APE values of identified model parameters for all cases of patient effort is much lower with a smaller interquartile range than the polynomial model [2] results. From Fig. 3(**a-d**) and Fig. 4(**a-d**), the fitted sine-wave model is able to model the forward simulated pressure profile well. Nevertheless, APE values for the identified Pstr is higher than E and R which is likely due to the sinusoidal function containing two Pstr terms. The SSE Contours in Fig. 4(**e-h**) show that the sine-wave model is practically nonidentifiable similar to the

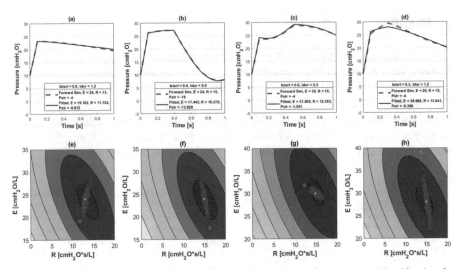

Fig. 4. Cases of successful sine-wave model fitting but unsuccessful parameter identification for breaths with patient effort. (*Top Row*) Plot of forward simulated pressure curve and the fitted sine-wave model. (*Bottom Row*) SSE contours for identifiability analysis of the respective cases above it. (Marker indications are described in caption of Fig. 3).

Table 2. APE table of identified parameters for Successful Cases 1, 2, 3 and 4 in Fig. 3.

Successful case	Absolute percentage error, APE (%)		
	E	R	P_{str}
1	1.0087 [0.4853 – 1.7370]	2.8922 [1.3987 – 5.1099]	5.8167 [2.6972 – 10.8075]
2	1.0618 [0.5324 – 1.7646]	1.5299 [0.7071 – 2.6945]	1.1758 [0.5308 – 1.9323]
3	0.9294 [0.4257 – 1.6046]	1.4002 [0.6666 – 3.5239]	0
4	1.1968 [0.5207 – 2.1235]	2.0294 [0.9455 – 3.5239]	2.3749 [1.1735 – 3.9908]

Table 3. APE table of identified parameters for Unsuccessful Cases 1, 2, 3 and 4 in Fig. 4.

Unsuccessful Case	Absolute Percentage Error, APE (%)		
	E	R	P_{str}
1	3.8530 [1.9620 – 6.4840]	2.0634 [0.9570 – 3.4888]	13.3970 [6.2195 – 22.5864]
2	4.4122 [2.1041 – 7.5579]	1.8031 [0.8707 – 3.1194]	3.1326 [1.4420 – 5.2785]
3	1.1501 [0.5652 – 2.0289]	2.8006 [1.2482 – 4.8521]	9.7681 [4.8038 – 18.2953]
4	6.0736 [2.9469 – 10.6387]	2.2672 [1.0328 – 3.8681]	20.9346 [10.2251 – 36.0857]

polynomial model [2]. However, the contours for the sine-wave model exhibit smaller confidence intervals [10, 17] than the contours of the polynomial model [2]. As such, the sine-wave model has a higher likelihood and consistency of identifying a distinct and unique solution [10, 17]. Most importantly, the sine-wave model is better suited for clinical application because the identifiable parameters are physiological (Pstr is the magnitude of patient effort) in comparison to the polynomial coefficients (a, b and c) in the polynomial model.

4.2 Successful Parameter Identification Cases

Upon conducting thorough investigation of all breath cycles in the Monte-Carlo Analysis, several successful cases of parameter identification are distinguishable. Generally, the sine-wave model performs well for patient effort that occurs during mid-breath and for a short period of time (Fig. 1) because minimal data is affected. Unique cases of successful parameter identification are presented in Fig. 3. Firstly, for patient effort that occurs before inspiration and creeps into the next inspiration cycle, the model is able to identify model parameters if there is sufficient unaffected data for the model to converge (Fig. 3(**a**)). Similarly, for patient effort which starts at the beginning of inspiration but for a short period of time, parameter identification is successful for all values of Pstr (Fig. 3(**b**)). These cases prove an improvement from the polynomial model which does not perform well in cases of early patient effort. Next, parameter identification is successful when patient effort occurs before inspiration but is not long enough to affect the subsequent inspiration cycle (Fig. 3(**c**)). There is no perturbation in the data, hence the single compartment model terms in the sine-wave model fits the affected waveform well. Finally, cases where patient effort occurs late during inspiration no matter short or long (Fig. 3(**d**)) results in successful parameter identification of E and R but not for Pstr. This may be due to insufficient sinusoidal data for the function to converge to a distinct solution.

4.3 Unsuccessful Parameter Identification Cases

Several cases where the sine-wave model performs less well have also been observed. These cases are similar to those described by Chee et al. [2] whereby E and R are misidentified if the patient effort alters the critical aspects of the pressure curve. The pressure due to resistance (R) component is dependent on flow and the pressure due to elastance (E) component is dependent on volume [2]. Thus, airway pressure is dominated by these components at separate times during inspiration due to the profile of flow and volume. Figure 5 below shows the relationship between flow and volume on the airway pressure. Resistance (R) influences the height and gradient of the inflection point where the straight line transitions into the polynomial curve. On the other hand, elastance (E) affects the height of the polynomial curvature.

The effects of these parameter dependencies are reflected as unsuccessful parameter identification cases if these traits are unable to be expressed. The first case of inconsistent parameter identification is for flat pressure profiles as a result of patient effort (Fig. 4(**a**), (**d**)). Certain combinations of model parameters can produce a flat curve which causes the model difficulty in identifying E as seen from the large confidence intervals in Fig. 4(**e**),

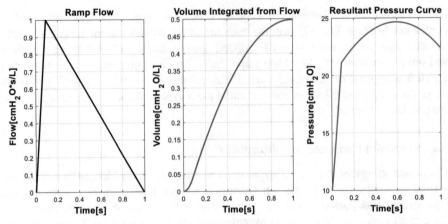

Fig. 5. Ramp flow profile (*Left*), volume profile (*Middle*) and resultant pressure profile (*Right*).

(**h**). As mentioned, the polynomial curvature is omitted, causing an inconsistency in identifying E. On the contrary, Fig. 4(**c**) shows a case where the inflection point is not expressed due to early and sufficiently long patient effort. In this case, the model has difficulty in identifying R proven by the large confidence intervals of R in Fig. 4(**g**).

Therefore, the sine-wave model is still limited for cases where the characteristics of the airway pressure is not sufficiently defined. This is due to the limitations of the single compartment model for spontaneously breathing patients. In addition, this study is still limited by the preset t_s and t_{dur} of patient effort. This continues to pose a challenge to researchers due to the amount of noise and erratic data in clinical data. Future work can be conducted with models without the single compartment model such as Bessel functions as well as determining a physiologically acceptable way of determining t_s and t_{dur}.

5   Conclusions

In conclusion, the sine-wave model as suggested by Redmond et al. [6] has been investigated in this study using the modified sine function from Vicario et al. [3] and referenced with the existing polynomial model research. Results show a significant improvement in model fitting and parameter identification in simulated data for the sine-wave model. The sine-wave model is practically nonidentifiable [10] like the polynomial model but has identifiable parameters that are more physiologically suitable than the polynomial model.

Acknowledgement. The authors would like to thank the Ministry of Higher Education Malaysia (MOHE) Fundamental research grant scheme (FRGS) (Ref: FRGS/1/2016/TK03/MUSM/03/2), Monash University Malaysia Advance Engineering Platform (AEP) and the MedTech Centre of Research Expertise, University of Canterbury for funding and support of this research.

Conflict of Interest. The authors declare that they have no conflict of interest.

References

1. Chiew, Y.S., et al.: Assessing mechanical ventilation asynchrony through iterative airway pressure reconstruction. Comput. Methods Programs Biomed. **157**, 217–224 (2018)
2. Chee, J.Z., Chiew, Y.S., Tan, C.P., Arunachalam, G.: Identifiability of patient effort respiratory mechanics model. In: 2018 IEEE-EMBS Conference on Biomedical Engineering and Sciences (IECBES), pp. 48–53 (2018)
3. Vicario, F., Albanese, A., Karamolegkos, N., Wang, D., Seiver, A., Chbat, N.W.: Noninvasive estimation of respiratory mechanics in spontaneously breathing ventilated patients: a constrained optimization approach. IEEE Trans. Biomed. Eng. **63**(4), 775–787 (2016)
4. Chiew, Y.S., et al.: Feasibility of titrating PEEP to minimum elastance for mechanically ventilated patients. Pilot Feasibil. Stud. **1**(1), 9 (2015)
5. Polese, G., Serra, A., Rossi, A.: Respiratory mechanics in the intensive care unit (2019)
6. Redmond, D., Docherty, P., Chiew, Y.S., Chase, J.: A polynomial model of patient-specific breathing effort during controlled mechanical ventilation (2015)
7. Akoumianaki, E., et al.: Mechanical ventilation-induced reverse-triggered breaths: a frequently unrecognized form of neuromechanical coupling. Chest **143**(4), 927–938 (2013)
8. Major, V., et al.: Respiratory mechanics assessment for reverse-triggered breathing cycles using pressure reconstruction. Biomed. Signal Process. Control **23**, 1–9 (2016)
9. Chiew, Y.S., et al.: Time-varying respiratory system elastance: a physiological model for patients who are spontaneously breathing. PLoS ONE **10**(1), e0114847 (2015)
10. Raue, A., et al.: Structural and practical identifiability analysis of partially observed dynamical models by exploiting the profile likelihood. (in eng). Bioinformatics **25**(15), 1923–1929 (2009)
11. Szlavecz, A., et al.: the clinical utilisation of respiratory elastance software (CURE Soft): a bedside software for real-time respiratory mechanics monitoring and mechanical ventilation management. BioMed. Eng. OnLine **13**, 140 (2014)
12. Schranz, C., Docherty, P.D., Chiew, Y.S., Möller, K., Chase, J.G.: Iterative integral parameter identification of a respiratory mechanics model. BioMed. Eng. OnLine **11**, 38 (2012)
13. Chiew, Y.S., Chase, J.G., Shaw, G.M., Sundaresan, A., Desaive, T.: Model-based PEEP optimisation in mechanical ventilation. BioMed. Eng. OnLine **10**(1), 111 (2011)
14. Drunen, E.J.V., Chiew, Y.S., Chase, J.G., Lambermont, B., Janssen, N., Desaive, T.: Model-based respiratory mechanics to titrate PEEP and monitor disease state for experimental ARDS subjects. In: 2013 35th Annual International Conference of the IEEE Engineering in Medicine and Biology Society (EMBC), pp. 5224–5227 (2013)
15. Chatburn, R.L.: Understanding mechanical ventilators. Expert Rev. Respirat. Med. **4**(6), 809 (2010)
16. Kroese, D.P., Brereton, T., Taimre, T., Botev, Z.I.: Why the Monte Carlo method is so important today. Wiley Interdisci. Rev. Comput. Stat. **6**(6), 386–392 (2014)
17. Raue, A., Becker, V., Klingmuller, U., Timmer, J.: Identifiability and observability analysis for experimental design in nonlinear dynamical models. Chaos **20**(4), 045105 (2010). (in eng)

Mask R-CNN for Segmentation of Left Ventricle

Muhammad Ali Shoaib[1], Khin Wee Lai[2(✉)], Azira Khalil[3], and Joon Huang Chuah[1]

[1] Department of Electrical Engineering, University of Malaya, Kuala Lumpur, Malaysia
shoaib.te@gmail.com, jhchuah@um.edu.my
[2] Department of Biomedical Engineering, University of Malaya, Kuala Lumpur, Malaysia
lai.khinwee@um.edu.my
[3] Faculty of Science and Technology, International Islamic University of Malaysia,
Negeri Sembilan, Malaysia
azira@usim.edu.my

Abstract. Globally, cardiovascular diseases (CVDs) remain the major cause of death among citizens. With echocardiography, doctors are able to diagnose and determine vital parameters for the evaluation of these diseases. Segmentation of left ventricular (LV) from echocardiography is a significant tool for cardiovascular medical analysis. Besides calculating important clinical indices (e.g. ejection fraction), segmentation also can be useful for the investigation of the basic structure of ventricle. Automatic segmentation of the LV has become a valuable means in echocardiography as we can achieve fast and accurate results and a large number of cases can be handled with limited availability of experts. The Convolutional Neural Networks (CNN) have shown outstanding outcomes for image classification, detection, and segmentation in numerous fields. Recently Mask Regions Convolutional Neural Network (Mask R-CNN) has emerged as a very good segmentation model. In this work, Mask R-CNN is proposed for the segmentation of LV. The Mask R-CNN model is first fine-tuned with Common Object in Context (COCO) weights and then the model is trained with our own data. The model first finds out the region of interest (ROI) in the image that contains the desired object i.e. LV. In the ROI, the model segment LV by generating the mask around it. The results demonstrated by the proposed method segments the LV accurately and efficiently with limited training data.

Keywords: Deep learning · Segmentation · Medical images · Left ventricle

1 Introduction

Cardiovascular diseases (CVDs) are one of the leading causes of deaths in developing countries. The World Health Origination (WHO) estimated that annually one-third of deaths in the world occur due to CVDs [1]. Heart diseases are caused by different reasons but mainly associated with diminished LV function. The LV segmentation is important for the assessment of LV function as it describes the ventricular volume, ejection fraction, wall motion irregularities, and myocardial thickness [2].

To analyze the heart and its LV, echocardiography is widely used technique. Being non-invasive, low-cost and non-ionization radiation, echocardiography makes its place

© Springer Nature Switzerland AG 2021
F. Ibrahim et al. (Eds.): ICIBEL 2019, IFMBE Proceedings 81, pp. 14–22, 2021.
https://doi.org/10.1007/978-3-030-65092-6_2

as the most frequently used technique for myocardial analysis. Doctors interpret these images manually which highly depends upon the expertise of clinicians or doctors [3]. For LV assessment mostly, the segmentation is performed manually. Manual segmentation is more time-consuming, labor-intensive and more-often the expert's proficiency affected by their work overload. It is highly beneficial to develop an automatic system for segmentation of LV.

In this study, we are focusing on developing an automatic LV segmentation tool based on CNN. CNN is a useful neural network used for image processing. In CNN few coefficients are used to extract the information from image compared to a simple neural network. In convolutional layer, the same coefficients are used across the different location of the image so CNN requires less memory. CNN's have had massive success in segmentation problems [3, 4]. For segmentation, CNN architectures are used without fully connected layers. This allows generating the segmentation maps for images of any size. Mask R-CNN, a model of CNN, is designed to perform segmentation task on natural images. As compared to existing work, we proposed the usage of Mask R-CNN for the segmentation of LV. Mask R-CNN has been used for natural image segmentation but its application in medicine is very new. Our results show that we can apply the Mask R-CNN for the segmentation of LV and it gave very good results.

The rest of the paper is organized as follows. Section 2 describes the existing literature and related work, Sect. 3 provides the methodologies adopted and development of the model. Section 4 discusses the results and finally, conclusions are drawn in Sect. 5.

2 Literature Review

There are different methods proposed by researchers for the automated segmentation of LV such as deformable models, statistical models, and machine learning models. For example, the authors in [5–7] proposed the deformable model approach for segmentation of LV. Deformable models require the initial position and shape of the model to be very close to the structure of desire object in the image. As good initialization is needed for deformable models, this makes automatic segmentation limited. Presently, the common initialization method of LV segmentation is manual or semiautomatic. Therefore, precise and automatic initialization technique is crucial for fully automatic LV segmentation.

Statistical models are built on the statistical figures from big labeled data. The statistical figures from the labeled data are modeled using parameters mostly based on contour borders and image textures information in the image. In the recent past, the active appearance model (AAM) and active shape model (ASM) have been used for the LV segmentation of echocardiography [8, 9]. In these approach initialization and assumption of shape model restrict automatic segmentation.

Unlike statistical and deformable models, machine learning approaches are not depending on the initialization and, the assumption of shape and appearance. In machine learning, the deep learning and more specifically convolution neural networks have attained great segmentation results in natural images [10]. Due to outstanding achievement in natural image segmentation, some recent works have been done on the application of LV segmentation using CNN. However, the main edge in natural image segmentation is the availability of a large amount of data while for the LV segmentation training dataset is limited. Therefore, limited researchers try to apply deep learning for the LV segmentation task.

Some research combined deep learning method and deformable model to segment LV on cardiac images. In these works, deep learning methods were employed to detect and categories the ROI of LV, and then another postprocessing method was used to make a final segmentation of LV. In [11], Luo et.al used CNN with the deformable model to segment LV from 3D echocardiography. CNN is used initially to find out ROI and then used Gradient Vector Flow (GVF) snack deformable model for the segmentation. As for deformable models, good initialization needed so this is achieved by using stack autoencoder technique. Other researchers have applied deep learning on 3D echocardiography along with the deformable model. Fully Convolutional Network (FCN) is applied for coarse segmentation 2D and deformable model is used for fine segmentation [12].

As labeling of data is a very time-consuming task so researchers also used some machine learning algorithm to label the data and train the network. This pre-trained network is used on manually annotated data. In [13], U-net architecture is used for segmentation of LV. Instead of manual annotation, LV is modeled as cubic Hermite spline methods and transformation of points to fit the spline on LV is done using a Kalman filter. They pre-train the network using labeled data which is annotated using Kalman filter and then use fine-tuning using manually annotated data. This method can reduce the amount of manual labeling, but here again, the overall method is depending upon another method i.e. conventional machine learning.

3 Methodology

In this research, we utilize a deep learning method for segmentation of LV, unlike other previous researches which have used other methods like deformable or simple machine learning with deep learning. Mask R-CNN architecture is a promising approach for image segmentation.

3.1 Dataset and Annotation

Echocardiography data of thirty patients is collected from the institution specialized in cardiovascular diseases. In this research, the apical 4 chamber (A4C) view is used for the analysis of LV. For training the neural network, we obtain echocardiography videos of twenty-five patients. Performance of the trained model was analyzed by using the test data of five different patients not used in training. LV is labeled using the Visual Geometry Group (VGG) annotation tool. VGG Image Annotator (VIA) is an open source annotation tool and used to describe and label a region in an image. We classified into two classes in the images i.e. background and left ventricle. The professionals from the medical field authenticate the labeled images.

3.2 Neural Network

The data set available for training included data of 25 patients since the data was not sufficient for training, thus it was compensated using transfer learning. First, we trained the model with pre-trained COCO weights. After that, we used our own data for training the model. Currently, the Mask R-CNN have been mostly used for the segmentation of natural images and have shown very good results. In larger part, Mask R-CNN has been driven by powerful CNN architectures, such as the Faster R-CNN [14] used for object detection and FCN [10] used for semantic segmentation.

In faster R-CNN, Region Proposal Network (RPN) a fully convolutional network is used to extract region proposals. Thus, RPN proposes regions with objects for further classification. The second stage, which is in core Fast R-CNN extracts features from each proposed region and do the classification and bounding-box regression.

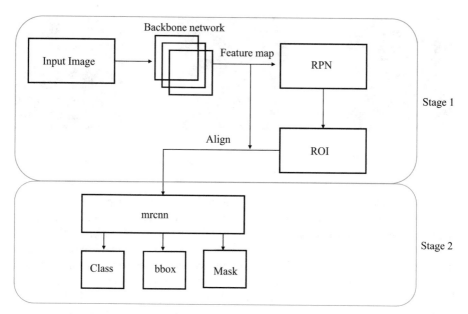

Fig. 1. Model Architecture

In the model of Mask R-CNN, we follow the same basic two-stage process of Faster R-CNN. In the first part backbone, neural network extracts the features from the image and passes to RPN and RPN extracts proposal regions. Here ROI-Align is used instead of ROI pooling to set the bounding boxes which could possibly contain the LV.

In the second stage, we not only predict the class and bounding box offset but also makes a binary mask for each ROI. Mask R-CNN works on the principle of faster R-CNN that applies bounding-box classification and regression in parallel. Fig. 1 shows the basic architecture of mask R-CNN. So, for each sample of ROI three losses are calculated: classification loss, bounding box offset loss, and mask loss.

$$L = L_{class} + L_{bbox} + L_{mask}$$

The neural network training was implemented using TensorFlow and Keras in NVIDIA DIGITS (GTX1080Ti) on an Intel Core i7. The learning rate of 0.01 and 50 epochs are used for training.

4   Results

In this paper, we present the initial results achieved by our proposed technique. Fig. 2(a) shows the one sample image of echocardiography images. In Fig. 2(b) LV boundary is drawn using the VGG annotator tool. These labeled images are used for training and testing. Fig. 2(c) is the output generated by the model. As Mask R-CNN has two stages, in the first part rectangular box is generated by RPN. The dotted line in the output figure shows the ROI generated by RPN. The second stage mask is generated within the ROI, the red labeled area is the segmented LV.

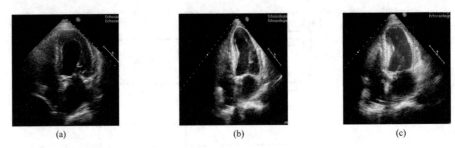

(a)   (b)   (c)

Fig. 2. (a) Echocardiography image (b) labeled image (c) segmented output

First, we will show some loss reduction during the training process. The losses during the training after each epoch have been analyzed. Tensorborad utility is used for analyzing the losses during training. Tensorboard is a remarkable utility which allows us to visualize data and how it behaves. The robustness of the neural network can be analyzed by the loss functions. The training process continued to 50 epochs. We use a smooth L1 loss, which is the absolute value between the prediction and ground truth. The reason is that L1 loss is less sensitive to outliers compared to losses like L2.

The model first calculates the Bounding box refinement loss. Figure 3 shows the bbox loss with the number of epochs on the x-axis. Loss decreases from 0.3505 to 0.0121 in 50 epochs.

The second loss is class loss. In this study, we have only two classes i.e. background and LV. The model calculates the class loss and Fig. 4 demonstrates the reduction in class loss with the number of epochs.

The model segments the LV and generates the mask of it. The mask loss is a loss of mask generated by the model and the original boundary of LV. In FCN mask loss is combined loss of mask and class of object, while Mask R-CNN only calculate mask loss here as the class has been already identified. Figure 5 represents the mask loss of the model that is 0.457 after first epoch and 0.057 after 50 epochs.

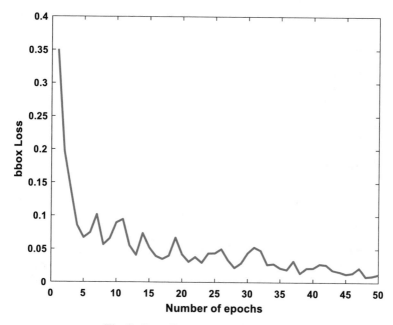

Fig. 3. Bounding box loss of the model

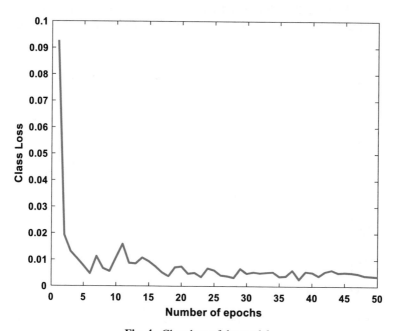

Fig. 4. Class loss of the model

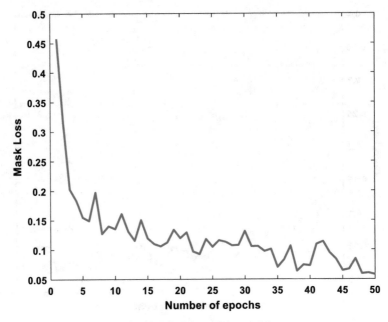

Fig. 5. Mask loss of the model

The overall loss function is calculated by adding all loss values like bbox loss, class loss and segmented mask loss. All these losses are shown in the above figures and overall loss is shown in Fig. 6.

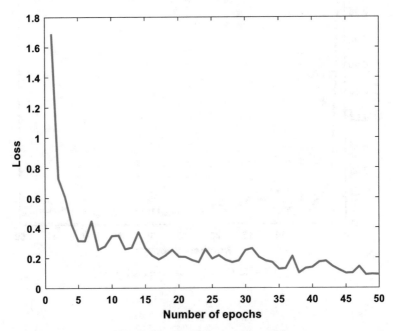

Fig. 6. The overall loss of the model

We also evaluate the segmented accuracy by using the Dice Similarity coefficient (DSC) [15, 16] It measures the overlap region between segmented and ground truth image using the following formula.

$$DSC = \frac{2|A \cup B|}{|A| + |B|}$$

DSC is equaled to the twice the number of pixels common in both ground truth and segmented binary masks divided by a total number of pixels in both marks.

We evaluate the model by calculating the DSC of all images of five patients. The data of these patients were reserved for the test purpose only and was not used for training, so all the data was unseen for the model before. The average value of DSC was 0.8940 ± 0.0365. Three examples of ground truth and segmented binary masks with DSC values are shown in Fig. 7.

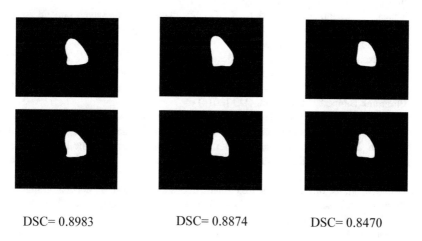

DSC= 0.8983   DSC= 0.8874   DSC= 0.8470

Fig. 7. Three samples of ground truth (top) and segmented binary masks (bottom)

5 Conclusion

This paper proposed a fully automatic method for LV segmentation using Mask R-CNN model. Our trained convolutional neural network first correctly detects the ROI and then generate the mask precisely. In case of lacking training data, we successfully applied to transfer learning by first training the network with COCO weights. DSC value shows that our results are very promising and encouraging. These experimental results proposed that the Mask R-CNN model on the area of nature image can be effectively transferred to the field of echocardiography images segmentation.

As future work, the authors plan to evaluate the model on other data sets to test the robustness and generality of the proposed approach. Effect of increasing the training data on the accuracy and losses of the model will be analyzed. Also, the evaluation of the model using different evaluation matrices and clinical indices will be done in the future.

Acknowledgement. This work was supported by Fundamental Research Grant Scheme (FRGS) FP092-2018A, Ministry of Education, Malaysia.

References

1. Saldivar, F., et al.: The worldwide environment of cardiovascular disease: prevalence, diagnosis, therapy, and policy issues. J. Am. Coll. Cardiol. **60**(25), S1–S49 (2012)
2. Sinusas, A.J., et al.: Contour tracking in echocardiographic sequences via sparse representation and dictionary learning. Med. Image Anal. **18**(2), 253–271 (2013)
3. Hanif, M., Nizar, A., Khalil, A., Chan, C.K., Utama, N.P., Lai, K.W.: Pilot study on machine learning for aortic valve detection in echocardiography images **8**(xx), 1–6 (2018)
4. Ibtehaz, N., Rahman, M.S.: MultiResUNet: rethinking the U-Net architecture for multimodal biomedical image segmentation, pp. 1–25 (2019)
5. Zhang, Y., Chandler, D.M., Mou, X.: Quality assessment of screen content images via convolutional-neural-network-based synthetic/natural segmentation. IEEE Trans. Image Process. **27**(10), 5113–5128 (2018)
6. de Alexandria, A.R., Cortez, P.C., Bessa, J.A., da Silva Félix, J.H., de Abreu, J.S., de Albuquerque, V.H.C.: PSnakes: a new radial active contour model and its application in the segmentation of the left ventricle from echocardiographic images. Comput. Methods Programs Biomed., **116**(3), 260–273 (2014)
7. Dietenbeck, T., et al.: Whole myocardium tracking in 2D-echocardiography in multiple orientations using a motion constrained level-set. Med. Image Anal. **18**(3), 500–514 (2014)
8. Barbosa, D., Friboulet, D., Jan, D., Bernard, O.: Fast tracking of the left ventricle using global anatomical affine optical flow and local recursive block matching. Midas J.**10** (2014)
9. D'hooge, J., et al.: Real-time 3D interactive segmentation of echocardiographic data through user-based deformation of B-spline explicit active surfaces. Comput. Med. Imaging Graph.**38**(1), 57–67 (2013)
10. Shelhamer, E., Long, J., Darrell, T.: Fully convolutional networks for semantic segmentation. IEEE Trans. Pattern Anal. Mach. Intell. **39**(4), 640–651 (2017)
11. Luo, G., Zhang, H., Sun, G., Wang, K., Dong, S.: "A Left ventricular segmentation method on 3D echocardiography using deep learning and snake. 2016 Comput. Cardiol. Conf. **43**, 473–476 (2017)
12. Dong, S., Luo, G., Wang, K., Cao, S., Li, Q., Zhang, H.: A combined fully convolutional networks and deformable model for automatic left ventricle segmentation based on 3D echocardiography, vol. 2018 (2018)
13. Smistad, E., Ostvik, A., Haugen, B.O., Lovstakken, L.: 2D left ventricle segmentation using deep learning. In: IEEE International Ultrason. Symposium IUS, pp. 4–7 (2017)
14. Ren, S., He, K., Girshick, R., Sun, J.: Faster R-CNN: towards real-time object detection with region proposal networks. IEEE Trans. Pattern Anal. Mach. Intell. **39**(6), 1137–1149 (2017)
15. Khalil, A., Faisal, A., Ng, S.-C., Liew, Y.M., Lai, K.W.: Multimodality registration of two-dimensional echocardiography and cardiac CT for mitral valve diagnosis and surgical planning. J. Med. Imaging **4**(03), 1 (2017)
16. Khalil, A., Faisal, A., Lai, K.W., Ng, S.C., Liew, Y.M.: 2D to 3D fusion of echocardiography and cardiac CT for TAVR and TAVI image guidance. Med. Biol. Eng. Comput. **55**(8), 1317–1326 (2017)

Generative Adversarial Network in Reconstructing Asynchronous Breathing Cycle

N. L. Loo[1]($\boxtimes$) , Y. S. Chiew[1] , C. P. Tan[1] , G. Arunachalam[1] , A. M. Ralib[2] , and M. -B. Mat-Nor[2]

[1] Mechanical Engineering Department, Monash University Malaysia Campus, Bandar Sunway, Malaysia
{nien.loo,chiew.yeong.shiong}@monash.edu
[2] Department of Anaesthesiology, International Islamic University Malaysia Kuantan Campus, Kuantan, Malaysia
m.basri@iium.edu.my

Abstract. Asynchronous breathing (AB) during mechanical ventilation (MV) can have adverse effect towards a patient's recovery. Especially, the presence of AB will disrupt MV breathing profile; thus, misidentifying patient-specific condition. This paper demonstrates the ability of generative adversarial network (GAN) to reconstruct asynchronous breaths to a normal breath profile. The reconstructed clean airway pressure can provide better identification of patient's condition. A total of 120,000 asynchronous and normal breaths GAN training data set were simulated from a Gaussian effort model. The breaths consist of elastance from 15 to 35 cmH2O/L and resistance from 10 to 20 cmH2Os/L. Three GAN configurations were investigated in this study. The first GAN configuration trained with 120,000 breaths yielded error of median 6.0 cmH2O/L [interquartile range (IQR): 3.71-11.56]. The second configuration comprised of five GAN models improved with median error of 2.48 cmH2O/L [IQR: 1.19-4.69] with each model trained in five different elastance and resistance values. The third configuration had 15 GAN models with each model trained with one set of elastance and resistance. The median error was 0.70 cmH2O/L [IQR: 0.22-4.29] for the third configuration. The results indicate that by dissipating the classification task, the performance of GAN reconstructing AB can be improved. Realizing GAN in real-time to reconstruct AB to a normal breath can potentially improve patient's condition diagnosis.

Keywords: Generative adversarial network (GAN) · Asynchronous breathing (AB) · Machine learning

1 Introduction

Asynchronous breathing (AB) occurrence is prevalent during mechanical ventilation (MV) therapy, especially when the patient's natural breathing pattern is not synchronised with ventilator support [1]. The impact of frequent AB occurrence can be dire to patient

© Springer Nature Switzerland AG 2021
F. Ibrahim et al. (Eds.): ICIBEL 2019, IFMBE Proceedings 81, pp. 23–34, 2021.
https://doi.org/10.1007/978-3-030-65092-6_3

as it may cause dyspnoea, lengthen the patient's dependency on MV usage, increment sedative drugs usage and worsen mortality rate [1, 2]. Hence, it is important to monitor and adjust MV settings in the event of poor patient ventilator interaction (PVI) due to AB. However, adjusting MV to improve PVI is a challenging task for clinicians due to the heterogeneous patient's response to MV. Hence, clinicians often rely on experience and intuition to adjust MV based on observed PVI at the patient's bedside [3, 4].

The conventional method to quantify AB involves trained researchers eyeballing AB profile manually and retrospectively to compute asynchronous index (AI) [5]. Manual AB inspection is also arduous and impractical in a time-critical clinical environment [6, 7]. In addition, there is little to no research investigating into quantifying the magnitude of asynchrony. Thus, a method to quantify AB automatically in real-time is imperative and can potentially assist clinicians in improving MV delivery. There are several types of AB, such as flow asynchrony, delay and premature triggering, double triggering, ineffective triggering, auto triggering and reverse triggering [8], and each type of AB has unique patterns and shapes. Therefore, designing a model-based approach to quantify the magnitude for different AB types is difficult to achieve due to the presence of irregularities or anomalous patterns of AB airway pressure [9, 10].

In the literature, there were several methods proposed to measure the magnitude of AB. For example, Chiew et al. [11] proposed a mathematical model which is able to assess the underlying respiratory mechanics and quantify the magnitude of AB through reconstructing the asynchrony affected breathing cycle. However, the accuracy of a mathematical model to estimate patient's respiratory mechanics is highly dependent on the quality of measured data; inaccurate parameter estimation can occur any time due to the unpredictable occurrence of noise and changes in MV settings [9]. Akoumianaki et al. [12] have proposed to use esophageal pressure to monitor AB; however, this method often involves additional invasive measuring probe, costly, and potentially induce further stress to patients. Nonetheless, these methods aimed to determine the quality of PVI but unable to quantify the magnitude of individual AB.

This study presents a machine learning approach, Generative Adversarial Network (GAN) to reconstruct asynchronous breathing cycle to a normal breathing cycle for the use of quantifying the magnitude of AB. The principle of the approach is similar to Chiew et al. [11], where a model is used to reconstruct the breathing cycle for asynchrony magnitude quantification, but it does not rely on a set of mathematical equation. GAN is a machine learning technique comprises of two deep neural networks competing each other to generative modelling. During the training process, GAN will learn essential features or patterns in the data and mimic any distribution of data [13]. This method eliminates the need to explicit programming when designing an automated model to quantify the magnitude of AB.

2   Methodology

2.1   Simulated Data for GAN Development

In this study, 120,000 asynchronous airway pressure waveforms were simulated using a modified polynomial model [14], the Gaussian effort model. The elastance and resistance were set from 15 to 35 cmH2O/L and 10 to 20 cmH2Os/L. These synthetic breathing cycles with their ground truth (non-asynchrony cycle) were used for training of the GAN model. Each simulated breathing cycle consists of inspiration section and the data length of each breathing cycle is resampled at 51 data points. The magnitude of each breathing cycle was normalized to 0 and 1. Breathing cycles were saved in binary data format in Matlab format file (.mat). Figure 1 shows an example of a simulated AB with actual normal breathing cycle. Simulations were performed using Matlab R2018b (The MathWorks, Natick, MA, US).

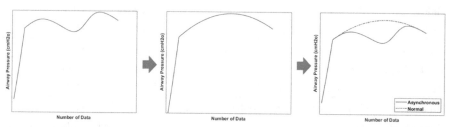

Fig. 1. Left: Simulated asynchronous breathing using Gaussian model. Middle: Normal breathing cycle with elastance of 25 cmH2O/L and resistance of 10 cmH20s/L. Left: normal and asynchronous breathing cycle.

2.2 Conventional Generative Adversarial Network

GAN is a class of deep learning technique which comprises of 2 neural networks competing with each other in a zero-sum game framework [13]. A GAN model consists of a generator G(Z) and discriminator D($\bar{x}$, T). The generator maps a random uniform noise sample, Z, as input and will learn to generate data or output a synthetic waveform, $\bar{x}$ similar to actual data points. On the other hand, discriminator will take $\bar{x}$ as output predictions to determine whether the output is close to the target. During training, D and G will contest with each other where G will minimize its action by generating a synthetic data which is similar to real data distribution, T; whereas, D will maximize its ability to determine the authenticity (real or fake) of the generated synthetic data. In that process, G will learn real data distribution and generate synthetic data similar to real data by computing the error, E. The objective function, J, of GAN can be expressed as:

$$\min_{G} \max_{D} J(D,G) = E\big[logD(\bar{x})\big] + E\big[\log(1 - D(G(Z)))\big]$$

Where E is the error computed by the discriminator or the generator. The output result of the discriminator is regarded as optimal when the distribution of the generated data is close or equivalent to the real data [13]. Table 1 and Fig. 2 shows the summary of the GAN architecture implemented in this study.

Table 1. Architecture of GAN model implemented throughout this study

	Settings/Name	Discriminator	
		Layer	Settings/Name
Input	51 x 1	Input	51x1
Activation	LeakyReLu (alpha = 0.2)	Convolution	32x3
Normalization	Batch Normalization (Momentum = 0.8)	Activation	Tanh
Hidden Layer	512 neurons	Dropout	0.5
Activation	LeakyReLu (alpha = 0.2)	Max Pooling	2
Normalization	Batch Normalization (Momentum = 0.8)	Convolution	32x3
Hidden Layer	1024 neurons	Activation	Tanh
Activation	LeakyReLu (alpha = 0.2)	Dropout	0.5
Normalization	Batch Normalization (Momentum = 0.8)	Max Pooling	2
Output layer	51 x 1	Hidden layer	128 neurons
Activation	LeakyReLu (alpha = 0.2)	Activation	Tanh
Normalization	Batch Normalization (Momentum = 0.8)	Output layer	1
		Activation	Sigmoid

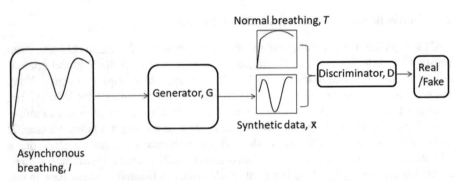

Fig. 2. GAN architecture during training. Asynchronous breathing will be the input of generator and discriminator will compare the generated x̄ data with ground truth, T.

2.3 Overview of the Model

The inputs, I for the generator are the simulated asynchronous breathing. The generator consists of 4 fully connected layers and 4 activation layers. Furthermore, to prevent overfitting, batch normalization is introduced to the output of all fully connected layers [15]. The generator will produce synthetic data, x̄ and passes the data to discriminator. On the contrary, discriminator will compare it with real data distribution T to compute the loss L to update the neurons in the networks during training. The discriminator architecture includes 2 convolutional layers, 4 activation layers, 2 fully connected layers and 2 pooling layers. Figures 3 and 4 show the generator and discriminator architectures.

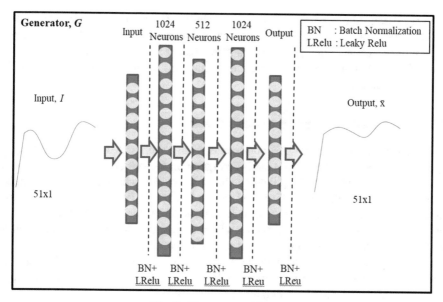

Fig. 3. Generator architecture

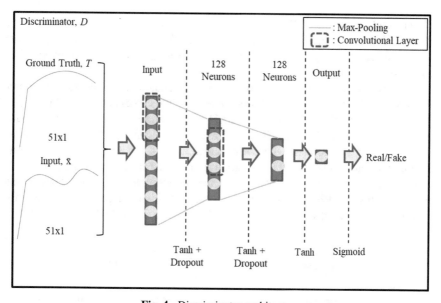

Fig. 4. Discriminator architecture

2.4 Computational Setup and Training Process

A Windows 10 computer with Intel Core i5-7400 CPU (4 cores), 32 GB DDR4 RAM and NVIDIA GTX 1050Ti 4 GB GPU was used for GAN training. All the models were trained offline in Python 3.5 (Python Software Foundation) and a python library,

Theano. Theano allows parallel computation using the Graphical Processing Unit (GPU) and it reduces resources and time needed in tuning the parameters. All of the models were trained 32 mini-batch size with adaptive moment estimation (Adam) as optimizer for 100 epochs. Batch normalization momentum was set as 0.8 and alpha value for LeakyRelu set as 0.2.

2.5 GAN Models' Performance and Evaluation

Performances of 3 different GAN configurations in restoring AB to normal breathing cycle were investigated. The first GAN configuration focuses on the performance of 1 GAN model, trained with 120,000 unique breathing cycles; whereas the second configuration had classification tasks dispersed among 5 GAN models. Each model dominant in five combinations of different elastance and resistance values. The third configuration had 15 GAN models, with each trained with only one set of elastance and resistance values. Figure 5 shows the configuration of GANs model in this study.

The respiratory mechanic parameter (resistance, R and elastance, E) values of each GAN reconstructed airway pressure, Paw_{gen} was estimated by fitting the single compartment model equation using linear regression [16]:

$$Paw_{gen} = RQ + EV + PEEP$$

In this study, airway flow, Q, and lung volume, V were kept constant and Positive End-Expiratory Pressure (PEEP) was kept as zero. 10,000 samples were randomly selected from the 120000 training dataset and used to validate against the performance of the trained models.

The performance of every GAN models was evaluated and compared using commonly used performance metrics such as Mean Absolute Percentage Error (MAPE) and Sum Squared Error (SSE). We assessed GAN performances by analysing the disparity between the generated elastance, Egen and resistance, Rgen with the actual elastance, Eac and resistance, Rac using the performance metrics. These performance metrics provided additional and detailed information for GAN performance evaluation.

MAPE measured the mean absolute distance between actual and predicted points. The non-negative MAPE characteristic promotes or facilitates aggregation of point distances over the data set in percentage [17]. Formula to compute MAPE is shown as below:

$$MAPE = Mean \left[\frac{(RM_{Actual} - RM_{GAN})}{RM_{Actual}} \right] \times 100\%$$

SSE, emphasizes or penalizes large errors (e > 1) but rewards or diminishes relatively small errors (e < 1). Thus, information from squared errors reflects the stability between synthetic data and actual data; hence, can potentially help us to facilitate optimization due to the simplicity of the analysis [18]. The SSE formula is shown as below:

$$SSE = (RM_{Actual} - RM_{GAN})^2$$

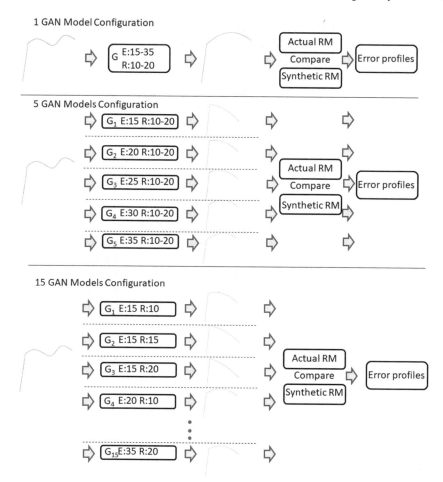

Fig. 5. 3 different GANs configuration.

3   Results

The results show that, GAN successfully identified the patterns of asynchronous breathing cycle and was able to recreate a normal breathing cycle that of the asynchronous cycle. Figure 6(a–b) shows 2 successfully reconstructed airway pressure using GAN as the generated airway pressure intimately resembles the actual airway pressure with minimal error (MAPE = 2.4% (Fig. 6a), 3.0% (Fig. 6b) and SSE = 338.4 (Fig. 6a), 105.2 (Fig. 6b)). The absolute error between Egen and Eactual were 0.91 (Fig. 6a) and 0.88 (Fig. 6b) cmH2O/L and Rgen and Ractual were 0.14 (Fig. 6a) and 0.04 (Fig. 6b) cmH2Os/L.

Figures 7 and 8 show the SSE and MAPE empirical cumulative distribution plot for all GAN configurations. The summaries of SSE and MAPE for all GAN configurations were shown in Tables 2 and 3. The 1 GAN model configuration yields the highest error with 8.36 cmH2O/L and 3.27 cmH2Os/L. 5 GAN models configuration achieved median error of 2.48 cmH2O/L [IQR: 1.19-4.69] and 1.32 cmH2Os/L [0.60 - 3.63]. For 15 GAN models configuration, the median error was 0.70 cmH2O/L [IQR: 0.22-4.29] and 0.25 cmH2Os/L [IQR: 0.12-0.46].

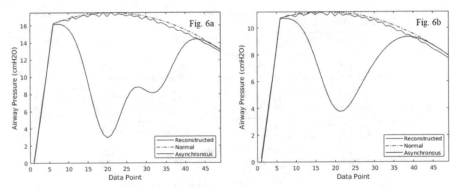

Fig. 6. Comparison of GAN reconstructed airway pressure and actual normal airway pressure when given AB as input when using 1 GAN model configuration. The generated airway pressure agrees the features defining a normal breathing cycle but with the presence of small magnitude noises.

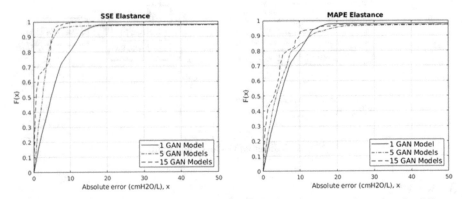

Fig. 7. Empirical cumulative distribution plot of different GAN model configurations by different performance metrics

Table 2. Results of performance metrics for GANs with different configurations when evaluating elastance value

Configuration	SSE Median[IQR]	MAPE Median[IQR]
1 GAN model	4.71 [2.09-8.36]	4.71 [2.09-8.36]
5 GAN models	2.39 [1.04-3.68]	3.61 [1.31-7.00]
15 GAN models	0.70 [0.22-4.29]	3.03 [0.45-5.21]

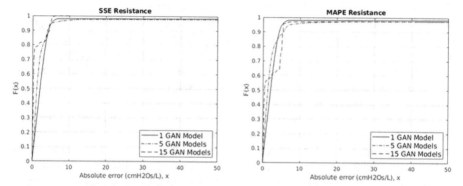

Fig. 8. Empirical cumulative distribution plot of the resistance absolute error when assessed with different performance metrics.

Table 3. Results of performance metrics for GANs with different configurations when evaluating resistance value

Configuration	SSE Median[IQR]	MAPE Median[IQR]
1 GAN model	2.08[1.03-3.27]	2.08[1.03-3.27]
5 GAN models	1.21[0.70-2.30]	1.35[0.62-2.47]
15 GAN models	0.25[0.12-0.46]	0.41[0.24-4.80]

4 Discussion

Tables 2 and 3 show that, the median SSE and MAPE decreased as the recognition and reconstruction tasks were distributed to more GAN models. It was found that the performance of 1-GAN model configuration was comparatively lower than the others. The higher errors in SSE and MAPE suggested that 1-GAN failed to capture and discriminate the essential asynchrony feature from different sets of breathing cycles. Figure 9 shows 2 cases where GAN fail to reconstruct a normal breathing cycle with MAPE = 49.5% (Fig. 9a), 25.9% (Fig. 9b) and SSE = 522.7 (Fig. 9), 1270 (Fig. 9b)). It is possible that the

ability to extract features in the GAN generator is hindered, resulting in lower GAN performance. In these cases, convolutional layers that can convolve inputs to determine the
relationship between data points for features extraction can be implemented to improve
the learning and resembling data distribution performances [19]. The performance of
5-GAN models configuration was better when it is tasked to detect a smaller range of
elastance and resistance values. This implied that the GAN model is able to achieve
better result when the training dataset is reduced. Specifically, to avoid overfitting or
'confuses' GAN when learning high similarities and indistinct patterns.

In this study, we demonstrated that GAN model is capable of learning and identifying
asynchronous breathing and reconstruct to a normal MV profile. The reconstructed normal airway pressure profile allows clinicians to better estimate the underlying respiratory
mechanics of the patient [20, 21]. The GAN's ability to recreate breathing cycle improved
when the classification tasks were dispersed to multiple GANs, however, the feasibility to deploy arbitrary number of models to detect and reconstruct a normal breathing
cycle clinically remains a concerned. Further investigation on 1-model GAN training
with additional data and different architecture is required to optimize the performance
of GAN to recognize and reconstruct asynchronous breathing cycles.

There are several notable works involving GAN in imagery and medical field. For
example, Reed et al. [22] demonstrated the technique to generate images from text
descriptions using GAN. Iqbal et al. [23] proposed the technique to generate realistic looking retinal images for supervised machine learning applications. Fei et al. [24]
implemented GAN to generate synthetic electrocardiogram (ECG) data that concede
actual clinical data while retaining and agreeing the features of patients with heart diseases. Thus, there is a growing interest in utilizing GAN in medical monitoring. The
GAN configurations presented in this study shows the potential of GAN being applied
in medical MV monitoring. The GANs are adept in extracting and learning essential features of MV breathing waveforms and recreating sensible outputs without supervision.

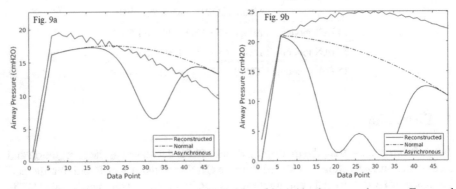

Fig. 9. GAN fail to reconstruct to actual normal breathing. Absolute error between Egen and
Eactual were 9.56 (Left) and 15.11 (Right) cmH2O/L. Absolute error between Rgen and Ractual
were 2.36 (left) and 4.29 (Right) cmH2Os/L.

5 Conclusion

In this paper, the performance of different GAN models in reconstructing a normal breathing cycle when given an augmented breathing cycle were investigated. The results showed that GAN was able to recreate normal breathing cycle with low error. However, additional studies are required to fully understand GANs limitation and feasibility in the mechanical ventilation monitoring.

Acknowledgement. The authors would like to thank the Ministry of Higher Education Malaysia (MOHE) Fundamental research grant scheme (FRGS) (Ref: FRGS/1/2016/TK03/MUSM/03/2), Monash University Malaysia Advance Engineering Platform (AEP), MedTech Core University of Canterbury for supporting this research.

References

1. Mellott, K.G., et al.: Patient ventilator asynchrony in critically ill adults: frequency and types (in eng). Heart Lung: J. Crit. Care **43**(3), 231–243 (2014)
2. Blanch, L., et al.: Asynchronies during mechanical ventilation are associated with mortality (in eng). Intensive Care Med. **41**(4), 633–641 (2015)
3. Brower, R.G., Matthay, M.A., Morris, A., Schoenfeld, D., Thompson, B.T., Wheeler, A.: Ventilation with lower tidal volumes as compared with traditional tidal volumes for acute lung injury and the acute respiratory distress syndrome (in eng), no. 0028-4793 (Print) (2000)
4. Brower, R.G., et al.: Higher versus lower positive end-expiratory pressures in patients with the acute respiratory distress syndrome (in eng), no. 1533-4406 (Electronic)
5. Bulleri, E., Fusi, C., Bambi, S., Pisani, L.: Patient-ventilator asynchronies: types, outcomes and nursing detection skills. Acta Bio Medica Atenei Parmensis **89**(7-S), 6–18 (2018)
6. Chao, D.C., Scheinhorn, D.J., Stearn-Hassenpflug, M.: Patient-ventilator trigger asynchrony in prolonged mechanical ventilation (in eng). Chest **112**(6), 1592–1599 (1997)
7. de Wit, M.: Monitoring of patient-ventilator interaction at the bedside. Respir. Care **56**, 61–72 (2011)
8. Mellott, K.G., et al.: Patient ventilator asynchrony in critically ill adults: frequency and types. Heart Lung **43**(3), 231–243 (2014)
9. Schranz, C., Docherty, P.D., Chiew, Y.S., Chase, J.G., Moller, K.: Structural identifiability and practical applicability of an alveolar recruitment model for ARDS patients (in eng). IEEE Trans. Biomed. Eng. **59**(12), 3396–3404 (2012)
10. Docherty, P.D., Schranz, C., Chiew, Y.-S., Möller, K., Chase, J.G.: Reformulation of the pressure-dependent recruitment model (PRM) of respiratory mechanics. Biomed. Sig. Process. Control **12**, 47–53 (2014)
11. Chiew, Y.S., et al.: Assessing mechanical ventilation asynchrony through iterative airway pressure reconstruction. Comput. Methods Programs Biomed. **157**, 217–224 (2018)
12. Akoumianaki, E., et al.: The application of esophageal pressure measurement in patients with respiratory failure (in eng). Am. J. Respir. Crit. Care Med. **189**(5), 520–531 (2014)
13. Goodfellow, I., et al.: Generative adversarial nets. In: Advances in Neural Information Processing Systems, pp. 2672–2680 (2014)
14. Redmond, D., Chiew, Y.S., Major, V., Chase, J.: Evaluation of model-based methods in estimating respiratory mechanics in the presence of variable patient effort (2016)
15. Ioffe, S., Szegedy, C.: Batch normalization: accelerating deep network training by reducing internal covariate shift. arXiv preprint arXiv:1502.03167 (2015)

16. Chiew, Y.S., et al.: Feasibility of titrating PEEP to minimum elastance for mechanically ventilated patients (in eng). Pilot Feasibility Stud. **1**, 9 (2015)
17. "MAPE (Mean Absolute Percentage Error) Mean Absolute Percentage Error (MAPE)". In: Swamidass, P.M. (ed.) Encyclopedia of Production and Manufacturing Management, p. 462. Springer US, Boston (2000)
18. Willmott, C.J., Matsuura, K.: Advantages of the Mean Absolute Error (MAE) over the Root Mean Square Error (RMSE) in Assessing Average Model Performance, p. 79 (2005)
19. Szegedy, C., et al.: Going deeper with convolutions. In: 2015 IEEE Conference on Computer Vision and Pattern Recognition (CVPR), pp. 1–9 (2015)
20. Damanhuri, N.S., et al.: Assessing respiratory mechanics using pressure reconstruction method in mechanically ventilated spontaneous breathing patient. Comput. Methods Programs Biomed. **130**, 175–185 (2016)
21. Major, V., et al.: Respiratory mechanics assessment for reverse-triggered breathing cycles using pressure reconstruction. Biomed. Sig. Process. Control **23**(Suppl. C), 1–9 (2016)
22. Reed, S., Akata, Z., Yan, X., Logeswaran, L., Schiele, B., Lee, H.: Generative Adversarial Text to Image Synthesis. arXiv.org (2016)
23. Iqbal, T., Ali, H.: Generative Adversarial Network for Medical Images (MI-GAN) (2018)
24. Zhu, F., Fei, Y., Fu, Y., Liu, Q., Shen, B.: Electrocardiogram generation with a bidirectional LSTM-CNN generative adversarial network (2019)

Modelling Patient's Spontaneous Effort During Controlled Mechanical Ventilation Using Basis Functions

Ganesa Ramachandran Arunachalam[1(✉)], Yeong Shiong Chiew[1], Chee Pin Tan[1], Azrina Mohd Ralib[2], and Mohd Basri Mat Nor[2]

[1] Monash University Malaysia, 47500 Bandar Sunway, Malaysia
{Ganesaramachandran.Arunachalam,Chiew.Yeong.Shiong, Tan.chee.pin}@monash.edu
[2] Kulliyah of Medicine, International Islamic University Malaysia Medical Center, Pahang, Malaysia
drazrina@gmail.com, basri.matnor@gmail.com

Abstract. During mechanical ventilation (MV) of respiratory failure patients, clinicians require real time patient-specific lung condition to set MV treatment. Application of mathematical models to determine patient-specific condition in setting MV is increasingly sought after amongst clinicians. However, when the patient is breathing spontaneously during controlled ventilation modes, estimation of respiratory mechanics becomes erroneous due to presence of patient inspiratory effort. Thus, there is a need to determine patient's respiratory mechanics during the presence of these efforts. This study presents a mathematical expression built on the single compartment model to determine patient respiratory mechanics. The model uses basis function and takes patient inspiratory effort into account. Inspiratory efforts of 1125 cases were simulated to determine the model performance and its stability. The study revealed that the model was capable of estimating asynchronous airway pressure. The model can be potentially useful to simulate any nonlinear airway pressure waveform with spontaneous effort.

Keywords: Mechanical ventilation · Respiratory mechanics model · Inspiratory effort

1 Introduction

Mechanical ventilation (MV) is an essential treatment for patients suffering from respiratory failure diseases [1]. These critically ill patients are supported by MV, by providing adequate air to maintain oxygenation and retain airway pressure [2, 3]. During MV, patients may breathe spontaneously with the support of controlled MV, but the patients' breath is sometimes not synchronous with the ventilator. Such asynchronous event potentially leads to inadequate oxygenation, ventilator associated lung injury and other cardiovascular complications [2, 3].

Application of mathematical models is increasingly sought-after amongst clinicians in setting MV therapy [4]. These models estimate patient-specific respiratory mechanics

© Springer Nature Switzerland AG 2021
F. Ibrahim et al. (Eds.): ICIBEL 2019, IFMBE Proceedings 81, pp. 35–45, 2021.
https://doi.org/10.1007/978-3-030-65092-6_4

using bedside-available MV data [5]. Numerical estimation of respiratory mechanics can assist clinician to diagnose respiratory failure disease, assess the effects of treatments and thus, adjust the ventilator settings to the patient specific need to improve MV delivery. Respiratory mechanics of the patient can be determined by fitting the MV data with mathematical models using least squares method. The well-known model used to estimate the respiratory mechanics of the patient is the *single compartment model* [4, 6]. The main limitation of this model is it does not consider the pressure generated by respiratory muscle during spontaneous breathing. Figure 1 shows airway pressure without effort and with effort. The change of airway pressure profile is evident when inspiratory effort is present as shown in the right sub-figure.

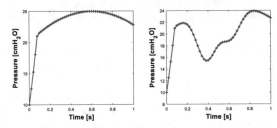

Fig. 1. Airway pressure waveform without patient effort (left), with patient effort (right)

The model presented in this paper, which is the *Gaussian effort model (GEM)* extends the conventional single compartment model using basis functions to estimate breath-by-breath respiratory mechanics of spontaneous breathing MV patients during volume-controlled mode. A Gaussian basis function is used to determine the complex shape of breath-specific patient effort [7]. The basis function assumes that the patient effort pressure is a linear combination of the sum of three simpler Gaussian basis functions as shown in Fig. 2. Basis function works in a similar manner to bases such as x-y coordinates that compose vector spaces in linear algebra. For instance, any vector in the two-dimensional coordinate system can be composed of linear combinations of x- and y-basis vectors. The basis vectors are linearly independent [7]. The basis function introduced in this paper potentially captures all patient effort features.

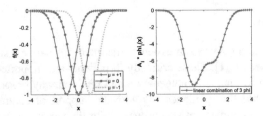

Fig. 2. Three separate Gaussian curves with different centroids (left). Sum of three separate Gaussian curves after multiplying each by appropriate constants (right)

In this study, simulated MV data were used to investigate the model's performance and clinical feasibility. The model was then further tested in real MV patient data who exhibit spontaneous effort during controlled ventilation. The success of this model not only helps to assess the patient-specific inspiratory effort but also enables the quantification of the mismatch between the machine and the man during MV therapy.

2 Method

The simulated airway pressure was generated initially with fixed values of E, R and airflow Q to test the Gaussian effort model. The E, R values calculated using Gaussian effort model is expected to be same as initially fixed values.

Then, the retrospective study was done using real patient data and the E, R values calculated using Gaussian effort model was compared with E, R values of Pressure reconstruction model [8] to verify the model accuracy. Pressure reconstruction model reconstructs effort free airway pressure using iterative method to estimate E, R [8].

2.1 Gaussian Model

Based on the observation of airway pressure waveform in clinical data, the shape of the patient's spontaneous effort during controlled ventilation is nonlinear. A linear combination of three Gaussian function is added to the single compartment model as patient effort $P_e(t)$ to represent the non-linear shape of patient effort. Then, the conventional single compartment lung model is revised to include a patient effort function $P_e(t)$. The Single compartment model is first defined as,

$$P_{aw}(t) = EV(t) + RQ(t) + P_0 \tag{1}$$

where P_{aw} is airway pressure, E is respiratory system elastance, R is respiratory system resistance, V is inspired volume, Q is air flow and P_0 is offset pressure [4, 6].

The basis function for patient effort is a function of pressure and it is denoted as,

$$P_e(t) = \sum_{i=1}^{3} A_i \emptyset_i, \ t_s \leq t \leq t_f \tag{2}$$

where,

$$\emptyset_i = e^{-\left(\frac{x-\mu_i}{\sigma_i}\right)^2} \tag{3}$$

$\emptyset_i$ represents the basis function, A_i represents peak effort pressure of ith Gaussian curve, μ_i and σ_i represents center and width of ith Gaussian curve respectively. Adding $P_e(t)$ into Eq. 1, the final Gaussian effort model (GEM) equation yield,

$$P_{aw}(t) = EV(t) + RQ(t) + P_0 + P_e(t) \tag{4}$$

where,

$$P_e(t) = \begin{cases} 0, \ t \leq t_s \\ \sum_{i=1}^{3} A_i e^{\left[-(x-\mu_i)^2\right]}, \ t_s \leq t \leq t_f \\ 0, \ t \geq t_f \end{cases} \tag{5}$$

where, $\mu_1 = -1$, $\mu_2 = 0$ and $\mu_3 = 1$, t_s and t_f denotes effort start time and finish time respectively. Equation 4 can be rewritten in matrix form as Eq. 6.

$$\left[V(t) \; Q(t) \; \emptyset_1(t) \; \emptyset_2(t) \; \emptyset_3(t) \right] \cdot \begin{bmatrix} E \\ R \\ A_1 \\ A_2 \\ A_3 \end{bmatrix} = [P(t) - P_0] \tag{6}$$

Equation 6 can be solved using nonlinear regression to find the values of parameters E, R, A_1, A_2 and A_3.

2.2 Simulation

A simulation was conducted to generate airway pressure and flow data using MATLAB R2018b (The Mathworks, Natick, Massachusetts, USA). In order to simulate and generate airway pressure, P_{aw} data, the following parameters were fixed initially, a) Flow was initially fixed at 0.5 L/s and then it was decreased gradually till zero till 1 s, creating a ramp flow profile. P_0 was set at 10 cmH2O; Elastance (E) and Resistance (R) were fixed at 25 cmH2O/L and 10 cmH2Os/L respectively.

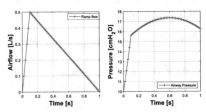

Fig. 3. Fixed ramp flow and corresponding airway pressure at set E 25 cmH2O/L and R at 10 cmH2Os/L

2.3 Model Fitting

The nonlinear least square solver function '*lsqnonlin.m*' in MATLAB is used to fit the basis function model. The following shows the sequence of the model fitting process.

Step 1: Model fit to original airway pressure to find patient effort timings
The original airway pressure is fitted to the single compartment linear lung model, Eq. 1, using the least square regression method [9]. Figure 4 shows the model fit with airway pressure data. The patient effort timings are determined by using fitting of the single compartment model to the original airway pressure.

Procedure to find t_s and t_f

Step a: The fitted model will have regions where the fitted pressure is higher than the original pressure. The area of these regions can be found by integrating the pressure difference over the regions. The largest region is taken as the patient effort occurring region. As shown in Fig. 3 fitted pressure is higher than original pressure between 'a' and 'b'. It is more likely that the patient effort occurs in this region and it is called "actual effort region". The start of the pressure effort is expected to be before the effort region i.e. point 'a' and the end of the effort will be expected after the region i.e. point 'b'.

Step b: The exact point of where effort starts is determined by finding the point of highest pressure before the actual effort region and similarly the exact point where effort finishes is located by identifying the highest pressure after actual effort region. As shown in Fig. 4, the highest pressure between point 'o' and point 'a' is taken as patient effort start time (t_s) and the highest pressure after point 'b' is taken as effort end time.

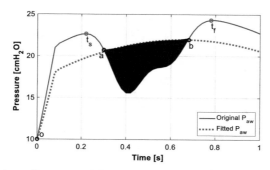

Fig. 4. Finding patient effort start and finish time by fitting single compartment model (dotted red). Black regions show where fitted pressure higher than original pressure. The region a-b is considered as patient effort region. Time at highest pressure before point a, and after point b are taken as effort start t_s and finish t_f time respectively

Step 2: Checking the presence of patient effort
After finding the region of effort, the area of the region is calculated. If the area of the effort region is less than 5% of the area under the original airway pressure curve, then the pressure is considered to be free of patient induced effort and the Gaussian model fitting will not take place and the respiratory mechanics will be estimated based on the single compartment model. 5% is a patient-specific threshold which can be changed in real time by clinicians.

Step 3: Separate and normalize patient effort
If the effort region area is more than the threshold, the effort pressure data is separated out and normalised to have the values between 0 and -1 to find the basis functions.
Step 4: Model fit to patient effort
After normalising, nonlinear least square fitting is done to patient effort data to find the parameters 'A_i' of normalized effort and 'μ_i' of the basis function $\emptyset_i$.
Step 5: Nonlinear fit to airway pressure

Finally, the original airway pressure is fitted with the GEM model as per Eq. 5 to identify E, R, A_1, A_2 and A_3.

2.4 Stability of Gaussian Effort Model

Monte-Carlo analysis was performed by altering different parameter values as mentioned in Table 1 to check the stability of the Gaussian model. Different airway pressure Profiles were generated by altering the parameters E and R of the single compartment model. Also, the range of different combinations of Gaussian model parameters such as μ, A_1, A_2 and A_3 were used to generate unique 1125 cases of patient effort. Randomly generated set of 5% noise were incorporated, with 1000 iterations for each cases, when generating pressure P_{aw} data to simulate noisy measurement (Fig. 5).

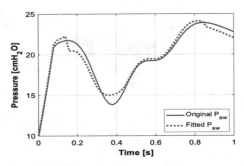

Fig. 5. Gaussian model fit to original airway pressure

Table 1. Range of parameters used in Monte-Carlo Analysis

Parameter	Range
E (cmH$_2$O/L)	15, 20, 25
R (cmH$_2$Os/L)	5, 10
A_1 (cmH$_2$O)	2, 4, 6, 8, 10
A_2 (cmH$_2$O)	2, 4, 6, 8, 10
A_3 (cmH$_2$O)	2, 4, 6, 8, 10
t_s (s)	0.12 ($\mu = -1$), 0.22 ($\mu = -1$), 0.3 ($\mu = -1$)
t_d (s)	0.42

2.5 Model Performance Evaluation

The model fitting of airway pressure is evaluated by calculating the absolute percentage error (APE) and sum of the squared error (SSE) between the estimated airway pressure by Gaussian model (P_{Fit}) and the original airway pressure (P_{aw}). The APE computes the percentage of deviation of model predicted values from preset values.

$$APE = abs\left(\frac{P_{Fit}(t) - P_{aw}(t)}{P_{Fit}(t)}\right) \times 100\% \tag{7}$$

$$SSE = \sum(P_{Fit}(t) - P_{aw}(t))^2 \tag{8}$$

The developed Gaussian model can be used to quantify the asynchronous breath also as it estimates the P_e separately. The peak patient effort P_{str} pressure can be determined for each breath as a metric to quantify the asynchrony.

2.6 Patient Data

Retrospective mechanically ventilated respiratory failure patients data were used to verify the Gaussian effort model. The data from ongoing CARE clinical observation trial in International Islamic University Malaysia Medical Center [10] is used. The patients were ventilated using a Puritan Bennett PB980 ventilator (Covidien, Boulder, CO, USA) with synchronous intermittent mandatory ventilation (SIMV) volume controlled mode. The clinical protocol and other details of the patient data used in this study can be found in the studies conducted by Chiew et al. [10]. CARE trial data composed of 10 patient data. 7 of 10 patients' data were used for retrospective analysis as they were ventilated with volume control mode. For each patient, 200 breaths with signs of spontaneous effort for each patient were analysed.

3 Result

The distribution of parameter combination, identified parameters and model fitting absolute percentage error and peak effort pressure P_{str} across 1125000 cases of patient effort are shown in Table 2. The overall absolute percentage error (APE) of fitted airway pressure is Interquartile range IQR: 4.7% [2.6–13.2]. The overall estimated P_{str} IQR 11.6 [12.9–15.1] cmH$_2$O.

Table 2. IQR of the APE of Fitted Paw, identified E & R

μ	E	R	APE of Paw	APE of E	APE of R	P_{str} set [cmH$_2$O]	P_{str} Cal [cmH$_2$O]
−1	25	10	3.08 [1.4–6.7]	4.6 [2.8–6.8]	5.86 [3.8–9.2]	10	12 [13.9–16.2]
0	25	10	2.7 [1.2–4.9]	4.89 [2.7–6.7]	3.76 [1.94–6.3]	10	11.4 [13.3–15.3]
1	25	10	2.05 [0.9–4.6]	4.31 [2.7–6.8]	2.81 [1.47–5.1]	10	10.32 [12.3–14.1]

The respiratory mechanics parameters of Gaussian model and Pressure Reconstruction model for all 7 patients are estimated as shown in Table 3. The absolute percentage error (APE) and sum of the square error (SSE) between Gaussian model and Single compartment model are shown in Table 4.

Table 3. IQR comparison of Gaussian model and Pressure reconstruction model parameters E & R

Patient	Gaussian model (GEM)		Reconstruction model	
	$E_{Gaussian}$ [cmH$_2$O/l]	$R_{Gaussian}$ [cmH$_2$Os/l]	E_{Rec} [cmH$_2$O/l]	R_{Rec} [cmH$_2$Os/l]
P1	33.5 [24.5–41.1]	7.9 [4.5–9.8]	33.9 [26.8–44.1]	7.6 [3.7–10.1]
P2	0.9 [0–11.3]	7.1 [1.9–8.9]	3.8 [1.7–10.7]	12.9 [10.8–14.8]
P4	21.1 [10.0–24.0]	8.2 [2.2–9.2]	26.8 [25.3–29.4]	4.3 [3.3–8.5]
P5	16.2 [9.2–31.5]	3.8 [0–7.1]	42.0 [35.3–45.5]	5.5 [− 0.5–8.3]
P7	32.2 [9.0–36.3]	7.7 [1.9–8.7]	35.1 [33.8–36.9]	7.7 [6.8–8.9]
P9	12.5 [8.3–35.9]	1.8 [0.2–5.9]	39.9 [33.1–45.4]	5.5 [−0.7–7.1]
P10	26.1 [14.0–44.5]	11.3 [6.9–15.4]	21.6 [10.3–46.9]	11.4 [7.1–20.8]
Median [IQR]	20.4 [10.7–32.1]	6.8 [2.5–9.2]	29.0 [23.7–36.9]	7.8 [4.7–11.2]

* $p < 0.05$ when comparing GEM and Pressure Reconstruction model using Wilcoxon-Ranksum test.

4   Discussion

The performance of a conventional single compartment model in capturing the respiratory mechanics of MV patients is poor when patient inspiratory effort is present. It is clear that there is a need of a better model to achieve good model fitting and representation. In this study, the model is extended by adding a basis function to capture inspiratory effort pressure to the single compartment model. The Gaussian model presented in this study is not only able to estimate respiratory mechanics of patient during asynchronous breathing but also can evaluate patient effort.

The model fitting error (APE) is less than 10% for entire 1 125 000 cases. This verifies that the developed Gaussian effort model works better for all simulated patient effort conditions and the model is capable of predicting the airway pressure

Table 4. IQR comparison percentage APE and SSE of Gaussian model & Single compartment model for 7 patient data

Patient	Gaussian model		Single compartment model	
	APE [%]	SSE	APE [%]	SSE
P1	2.46 [5.5–10.4]	9.26 [12.3–15.4]	8.73 [4.2–15.8]	12.63 [15.7–20.3]
P2	0.7 [1.7–3.7]	4.36 [5.16–6.8]	5.63 [2.9–8.8]	6.78 [8.5–11.1]
P4	0.81 [2.0–5.5]	4.15 [6.19–7.2]	4.24 [2.3–12.8]	8.28 [11.5–13.3]
P5	0.7 [1.7–3.7]	2.93 [3.52–4.1]	3.45 [1.8–9.8]	6.31 [7.2–10.1]
P7	0.32 [0.8–2.1]	2.85 [3.1–3.2]	1.65 [0.9–3.9]	4.5 [5.4-5.9]
P9	0.88 [2.1–4.5]	3.56 [4.17–5.4]	5.68 [3.2–13.2]	6.06 [7.5–11.8]
P10	0.71 [1.9–4.9]	4.37 [6.58–8.5]	9.28 [4.9–15.4]	9.59 [14.0–22.6]
Median [IQR]	0.94 [2.2–5.1]	4.49 [5.8–7.25]	5.5 [2.9–11.4]	7.7 [10.1–13.6]

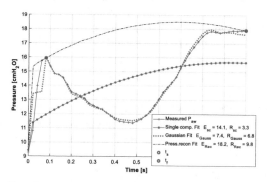

Fig. 6. Gaussian model fit to Patient 1 airway pressure data with effort

GEM model works well when the effort start t_s and finish time t_f is found precisely. Otherwise, the model fits to the original pressure very well but it could not estimate the parameters E and R accurately. The important criterion to achieve good prediction by Gaussian effort model is finding the exact timing of patient effort start (t_s) and finish. This can be done by having a discrete approach as follows. Single Compartment Model fitting is done, and the model and actual data intersecting points ('a' and 'b') are located to find the estimated effort start and finish time as shown in Fig. 4 step 1, 2, 3. As the perturbation due to inspiratory effort starts much before the first intersecting point 'a', the highest pressure point before point 'a' where the perturbation starts is taken as effort start time (t_s). Similarly, the perturbation due to effort ends much after the second intersecting point 'b'. The highest pressure point after point 'b' is taken as effort finish time. This method captures the entire perturbation region and considers it as patient effort region.

In this model, a set of three basic Gaussian basis functions is used as functional building blocks to design patient effort. After multiplying each Gaussian function by its own constant and summing it up, patient effort feature can be constructed to a single basis function. The linear combination of 3 Gaussian functions to model patient effort solves the problem of non-linearity.

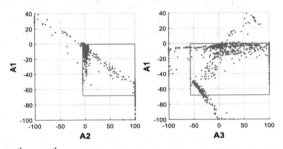

Fig. 7. 5th to 95th percentile of basis function magnitudes A_1, A_2 & A_3

The parameters such as E and R determined using Gaussian model were compared with the same that of pressure reconstruction model for validation. Table 3 shows the IQR of E and R for both models. It is found that the Gaussian model parameters and Pressure reconstruction model parameters have significant difference ($p < 0.05$) and the Gaussian model fails to capture the true respiratory mechanics. This is because during nonlinear regression all 5 parameters of Gaussian model (E, R, A_1, A_2 and A_3) have equal weightage which leads to underestimation of E and R. However, the Gaussian model is able to fit to the actual airway pressure better. As shown in Table 4, both the APE and SSE error of Gaussian model is lesser than the Single compartment model. As shown in Fig. 6, the Gaussian model fits very well with the actual data than any other model.

The 5th to 95th percentile of magnitude of the basis function A_1, A_2 and A_3 for all 7 patients for elastance range between 10 and 50 cmH$_2$O/L was shown in Fig. 7. These values $A_1 = -54.8$ [IQR: -11.71–4.51], $A_2 = -0.02$ [IQR: 2.92–100], and $A_3 = -37.22$ [IQR: -0.47–57.12], can be used to simulate any forms of patient spontaneous effort during controlled ventilation for further research.

5   Conclusion

In conclusion, the Gaussian effort model was presented to capture respiratory mechanics in the presence of patient inspiratory effect in volume control ventilation modes. The presented method is effective and robust not only to predict the respiratory mechanics but also to quantify the breath-specific asynchrony of patient and ventilator by estimating the peak patient effort pressure (P_{str}) separately. However, it was found that the accuracy of the estimated respiratory mechanics may vary when compared with the conventional Pressure reconstruction model. Nevertheless, the model is capable of having good fit and thus, it can be used to simulate any forms of pressure effort waveform.

Acknowledgement. The authors would like to thank the Ministry of Higher Education Malaysia (MOHE) Fundamental research grant scheme (FRGS) (Ref: FRGS/1/2016/TK03/MUSM/03/2), Monash University Malaysia Advance Engineering Platform (AEP) and the MedTech Centre of Research Expertise, University of Canterbury for funding and support of this research.

References

1. Marini, J.: Mechanical ventilation: past lessons and the near future. Crit. Care **17**(1), 1–10 (2013)
2. Gattinoni, L., et al.: Ventilator-induced lung injury: the anatomical and physiological framework. Crit. Care Med. **38**, S539–S548 (2010)
3. Brochard, L., Slutsky, A., Pesenti, A.: Mechanical ventilation to minimize progression of lung injury in acute respiratory failure. Am. J. Respir. Crit. Care Med. **195**(4), 438–442 (2017)
4. van Drunen, E.J., et al.: Model-based respiratory mechanics to titrate PEEP and monitor disease state for experimental ARDS subjects. In: 2013 35th Annual International Conference of the IEEE Engineering in Medicine and Biology Society (EMBC) (2013)
5. Chiew, Y., et al.: Feasibility of titrating PEEP to minimum elastance for mechanically ventilated patients. Pilot Feasibility Stud. **1**(1), 9 (2015)
6. Schranz, C., et al.: Iterative integral parameter identification of a respiratory mechanics model. Biomed. Eng. Online **11**(1), 38 (2012)
7. Simon, M.K.: Probability Distributions Involving Gaussian Random Variables: A Handbook for Engineers and Scientists. Springer, New York (2006)
8. Chiew, Y.S., Tan, C.P., Chase, J.G., Chiew, Y.W., Desaive, T., Ralib, A.M., Nor, M.B.M.: Assessing mechanical ventilation asynchrony through iterative airway pressure reconstruction. Comput. Methods Programs Biomed. **157**, 217–224 (2018)
9. Chiew, Y.S., et al.: Model-based PEEP optimisation in mechanical ventilation. Biomed. Eng. Online **10**(1), 111 (2011)
10. Chiew, Y.S., et al.: Clinical application of respiratory elastance (CARE trial) for mechanically ventilated respiratory failure patients: a model-based study. IFAC-PapersOnLine **51**(27), 209–214 (2018)

Anisotropic Diffusion for Reduction of Speckle Noise in Knee Articular Cartilage Ultrasound Images

Muhammad Ali Shoaib[1], Joon Huang Chuah[1], Azira Khalil[2],
Muhammad Hanif Ahmad Nizar[3], and Khin Wee Lai[3(✉)]

[1] Department of Electrical Engineering, University of Malaya, Kuala Lumpur, Malaysia
shoaib.te@gmail.com, jhchuah@um.edu.my
[2] Faculty of Science and Technology, International Islamic University of Malaysia,
Negeri Sembilan, Malaysia
azira@usim.edu.my
[3] Department of Biomedical Engineering, University of Malaya, Kuala Lumpur, Malaysia
mdhan1111@gmail.com, lai.khinwee@um.edu.my

Abstract. Ultrasound imaging is a very common imaging technique used for the analysis of knee osteoarthritis. Ultrasound imaging has numerous advantages over other available imaging techniques. It is a low cost, non-invasive, and non-ionizing radiation imaging technique. Beside these advantages of ultrasound, the two main drawbacks of ultrasound imaging i.e. low contrast ratio and speckle noise make it difficult to diagnose the cartilage shape of the knee joint. The aim of this paper is to present a technique for making diagnosis of cartilage easier by removing the speckle noise while preserving the edges in US image. This paper proposes a modified diffusivity function which can not only removes the noise but also preserves the edges. The performance of the proposed method is evaluated using peak signal to noise ratio and Equivalent Number of Looks.

Keywords: Diffusivity function · Speckle noise · Edge preservation

1 Introduction

Osteoarthritis (OA) in the knee joint is a dominant disease which affects the aged people. Progressive deterioration in the cartilage is one of the elementary reasons for this disease. According to some researchers 70 out of 100 people of sixty five years old have radiographic signs of OA [1]. To visualize the OA, different medical imaging systems like X-rays, magnetic resonance imaging (MRI), computed tomography (CT), and ultrasound (US) are typically used [2]. Most of these systems come with huge expenses or complexities. Among these, MRI is very expensive and not suitable for implanted patients. While CT not only releases a high level of radiation but also has a constraint for detecting a fracture. X-ray produces ionizing radiation and also lack in the description of soft tissue [3]. Unquestionably, all the said medical imaging methods have some drawbacks.

© Springer Nature Switzerland AG 2021
F. Ibrahim et al. (Eds.): ICIBEL 2019, IFMBE Proceedings 81, pp. 46–53, 2021.
https://doi.org/10.1007/978-3-030-65092-6_5

Consequently, US imaging looks like a valuable and useful method for knee OA assessment, especially in terms of cost, safety, and ease of use. In spite of having a lot of advantages, speckle noise and low contrast are two main demerits of US images. Hossain et al. in [2] work on issue of low contrast and enhance the contrast of US image. The second main problem with US image is speckles noise. The speckle noise is multiplicative noise [4]. It is produced due to the superposition of acoustic echo and generates a complicated interference pattern. This pattern is produced due to interference of US with the object of comparable size to sound wavelength. This speckle noise disguises the relevant information of the patient in the image. Hence, it is very important to retain the important detail of the original image by lowering the effect of speckle noise. For the reduction of speckle noise Anisotropic diffusion (AD) has been proposed years back [5]. The most important thing is to differentiate the gradient between edges and noise. Doing so, we can preserve the edge details of US image, but most of the AD methods cannot handle this problem efficiently and during the suppression of speckle they also lose the edges information.

In the current work, the focus is on reduction of speckle noise so that the joint cartilage images of knee US can be improved. The parameter settings of the AD filter, including gradient threshold, conductance or diffusivity function, and stopping criteria are discussed and improved. The performance of the method is examined by means of two different evaluation metrics. The real US images are used to apply the proposed method and to get the speckle free US images with sharp edges.

2 Literature Review

Noise in US images can be additive (Gaussian) and multiplicative (speckle). Removing speckle noise is significantly more difficult as compared to conventional Gaussian additive noise. This is because speckle noise signal is correlated, and its distribution is considerably more complicated than the Gaussian.

Perona-Malik in their work [5] suggested a new definition of scale space and proposed an algorithm based on AD. A nonlinear partial differential equation-based diffusion process is proposed by the authors. This technique is broadly used for image denoising. This method eliminated the demerits of linear smoothing i.e. the linear smoothing blurs the images and removes the significant detail but still edge preservation is compromised during noise reduction. A new technique Speckle Reducing Anisotropic Diffusion (SRAD) is proposed by Yu and Actor in [6]. They used a statistical method for suppression of speckle noise. In homogenous region isotropic diffusion is applied using non-linear filter to diminish the speckle and preserve the edges information, the diffusion process is stopped at the edges. In this way, this method attains stability in removing the speckle and preserving the edges. Even with this ability, SRAD is frequently incompetent to yield a suitable outcome in filtering US images.

The limitations of SARD are addressed by Laplacian Pyramid Nonlinear Diffusion (LPND) [7]. In this method the input image is decomposed into different sub-bands, a nonlinear diffusion process is performed to remove the speckle. Finally, the diffused Laplacian pyramid is reconstructed to get the despeckled image. Although LPND preserves edges while maximally eliminating speckle but the performance of this method highly depends upon the key parameters and results are hence its results are very much sensitive as they depend upon several key parameters. A denoising filter is proposed by Ling and Bovik [8] based on anisotropic diffusion. This method used the median filter in the diffusion step. Selection of image gradient threshold does not affect the filter which makes automatic image denoising easier, but the statistical characteristic of the speckle is not considered by this approach which degrades the robustness of the speckle reduction.

Based on the work of [9] Krissian et al. proposed Oriented Speckle Reducing Anisotropic Diffusion (OSRAD) in [6]. By revising the properties of SARD, this method used matrix diffusion equation. This method shows some advantage in reducing the noise and enhancing the edges but the overall the behavior and outcomes of OSRAD filter is almost same and parallel to that of the SRAD filter. Another method which focuses on calculating the coefficient of variation in noisy images is proposed by Aja-Fernandez et al. [10]. This method is named as Detail Preserving Anisotropic Diffusion (DPAD). This technique performs better than SRAD regarding a good estimation of the coefficient of variation, but it leads to over smoothing the image when a number of iterations are large. The improvement in PM is presented in [11] by Catte et al. In the noisy image, PM model generates an indistinguishable gradient of noise and image features. Catte et al. suggest that accurate parameter approximation is very important to efficiently implement the AD filter for noisy US images. As these parameters can preserve the edges speckle can be suppressed.

In reducing the speckle noise, the approaches mentioned earlier have limitations in edge preservation. So, there is a need to have an AD method which not only remove the speckle noise but also improve the performance of edge preservation.

3 Methodology

3.1 Data Acquisition

The data of US images of the knee joint was collected by scanning twenty healthy people by the professional sonographer. In the sample data, 60% of males and 40% of females' subjects are included. Two important sides i.e. medial and lateral sides of knee joints used for the precise observation of cartilage of knee joint. To get a good resolution image and detection of small imaging particles, the 8 MHz probe is used. The US machine used is "Aplio MX", manufactured by Toshiba.

3.2 Proposed Method

The diffusion Eq. (1) is used for our proposed method. This describes the diffusion model.

$$\begin{cases} \frac{\partial I}{\partial t} = div\big[g(|\nabla(G(\sigma) * I)|).\nabla I\big] \\ I(t=0) = I_0 \end{cases}, \tag{1}$$

In the above equation, I_0 is the original image. The standard deviation of pixels values is represented by σ, convolution operator is symbolized by symbol *, Gaussian filter in equation is denoted by G(.), and the convolution of image with Gaussian kernel is denoted by $G(\sigma) * I$. The divergence operator applied ion image is shown with div, and gradient operator which is used to calculate the change in intensity or color in any particular direction is symbolized with ∇, $\|$ compute the magnitude, and $g(|\nabla I|)$ denotes edge stopping function which stops the diffusion process at the edges of the image. This edge stopping function is also called a diffusion function. The equation was proposed by Catte_PM [12]. This model is used because it filters the high level of noise from the images efficiently.

To automatically compute σ associated with the Gaussian noise of the image, a window size of between 20 × 20 and 65 × 65 pixels is considered. Before calculating the final value of σ of Gaussian filter, first each block of different size is taken, and its standard deviation of each block is calculated. From these values the standard deviation of the most uniform block, σ of the Gaussian filter is measured. The size of the smoothing Gaussian filter is determined by using σ is explained in a study by Petrou et al. [13].

One of the main parameters in Eq. (1) is the diffusivity function. [14] in his work shows different diffusivity functions that differentiate the filtering results. Therefore, for the performance enhancement of the AD methods, it is significant to select a suitable diffusivity function. Furthermore, it should be scaled in a way so that it preserves the edge effectively. We proposed the diffusivity function based on the work of Black et al. in [14]. The diffusivity function is given by Eq. (2).

$$g(x) = \frac{1}{1 + \left(\frac{x}{k}\right)^2} \tag{2}$$

In Eq. (2) x represents the gradient and gradient threshold is represented by k. For effective edge detection, the parameter which have very active role is gradient threshold. If the gradient threshold is underestimated, then the model does not remove the noise effectively and hence it weakens the noise reduction ability. In addition, the overestimation of the gradient threshold over-smoothed the image. Therefore, to preserve the edges and suppressing noise successfully an optimum gradient threshold selection is required.

For scaling the diffusivity function, we consider some basics of digital signal processing. In digital image processing, normally 256 quantization levels are used to digitize the brightness of the image. So, for a digital image, it can consider that digital 0 is equivalent to $0.5/256 = 0.002$. Generally, the subjective recovery of the image is used for image enhancement. Hence, the change in grey tone should be measured that eyes of human can perceive. For greyscale images with 256 levels, the human eye can differentiate only fewer than 2 to 3 levels of variations. Therefore, the numerical value of $0.002 \times 3 = 0.0060 \sim 1/(1 + (12.17)^2)$ can be considered. Based on this statement, our diffusivity function gets the following form.

$$g(x) = \frac{1}{1 + \left(\frac{12.17x}{k}\right)^2} \tag{3}$$

The discrete form of the model is given by (4)

$$I_{t+1}(s) = I_t(s) + \frac{\lambda}{|\eta_s|} \sum_{p \in \eta_s} g_k\left(\left|\nabla I_{s,p}\right|\right) \nabla I_{s,p} \tag{4}$$

In above equation, t is the iteration steps, gradient threshold is represented with k, the position of pixel in discrete 2_D grid is denoted by s, and g is the conductance function. While, the diffusion rate is controlled by the parameter $\lambda \in (0, 1)$, η_s denotes the spatial neighborhood 4-pixel of s. In PM model author used $\eta_s = \{N, S, E, W\}$, where N is North, S is South, E is East, and W is West neighborhood of pixel s. In our proposed model we use to calculate diffusivity for eight directions so in our case $\eta_s = \{N, S, E, W, NE, WN, WS, SE\}$, where NE is north-east, WN is west-north, WS is west south, and SE is south-east neighborhood of the central pixel s.

The symbol ∇ is gradient operator of continuous form. Moreover, it specifies a scalar and it is a distance between two consecutive pixels i.e. the neighboring (p) and center pixel (s) in every direction. Therefore,

$$\nabla I_{s,p} = I_t(p) - I_t(s) \ and \ p \in \eta_s = \{N, \ S, \ E, \ W, \ NE, \ WN, \ WS, \ SE\} \qquad (5)$$

This is an iterative process and is commonly conducted for a certain number of iterations. One of very important feature which highly effects the performance of AD methods is to terminate the diffusion process automatically. The Mean Absolute Error (MAE) proposed by Zhang et al. in [7] proposed a method called Mean Absolute Error (MAE) for the termination of automatic diffusion process. The MAE stopping criterion is very effective for US images and therefore is used in our proposed method.

3.3   Evaluation Metrics

For assessing the performance of the proposed technique, two performance metrics peak signal to noise ratio (PSNR) [15, 16] and Equivalent Number of Looks (ENL) [17] are used. PSNR computes the capability of speckle noise reduction from noisy images. Decibel (dB) is the commonly used unit for PSNR is. A higher value of PSNR indicates that high level of noise is removed from the noisy image. PSNR calculation depends upon Mean Square Error (MSE). MSE computes the square difference between two pixels of different images and then takes the average of all differences. The equation to measure the MSE is as follow.

$$MSE = \frac{1}{M \times N} \sum_{(i,j)=1}^{M,N} (I_t(i, j) - I_0(i, j))^2 \qquad (6)$$

Here, I_0 represents the original image and is I_t the filtered image. M are number of rows and the columns are denoted by N in the image. The term (i, j) is used to show the spatial location of the pixels. PSNR is calculated using the value of MSE by the following equation.

$$PSNR = 10 \log_{10} \frac{max(I_0)^2}{MSE} \qquad (7)$$

Equivalent Number of Looks (ENL) is another significant metric for computing the speckle noise reduction. It is calculated by using the Equation

$$ENL = \left(\frac{Mean}{Standard \ Deviation} \right)^2 \qquad (8)$$

A large value of ENL shows that model has removed the speckle noise efficiently. The ENL is calculated by applying this on regions of image and hence size of region of image effect the ENL value. Theoretically, a small region gives the smaller ENL value as compared to a large region. In this situation, the accuracy can be attained by dividing the image into the 25 × 25 pixel region and ENL value is calculated for each region. The Final value of ENL is calculate by averaging the all ENL values of small regions.

4   Results

In this paper, we proposed a method for speckle noise reduction. Fig. 1 (a) is the original US image of medial side of knee joint cartilage of a man. The output image after speckle noise removal is shown in Fig. 1 (b). It is clear from fig b that "V" shape cartilage layer is very clear. Hence the proposed method removes the speckle noise and edges are also preserved.

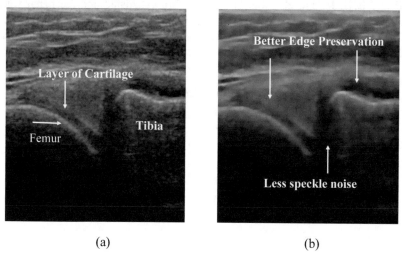

(a)   (b)

Fig. 1. Medial side of knee joint cartilage (a) original image. (b) AD filtered image using the proposed method

Similarly, Fig. 2 (a) shows the original lateral side of knee joint cartilage. Fig. 2 (b) represents the speckle free image after passing to the model. Fig. 2 (b) shows that "U" shape cartilage is reserved. As a result, it can be concluded that, with the help proposed diffusivity function, our method perform very good in edge preservation while reducing the speckle noise.

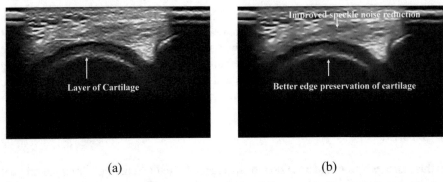

(a)   (b)

Fig. 2. Lateral side of knee joint cartilage (a) original image (b) AD filtered image by using the proposed method.

We also evaluate the output by calculating the PSNR and ENL of our images. The PSNR and ENL for the 20 subjects (healthy) are calculated and the mean value of results are represented in Table 1. The highest values of PSNR and ENL attain are 31.409 ± 1.031 and 30.297 ± 0.511 respectively. Our proposed method has considerably higher numerical values of the performance metrics.

Table 1. Mean and standard deviation value of PSNR and ENL

Evaluation metric	Mean ± SD	95% confidence interval of the difference	
		Lower bound	Upper bound
PSNR	31.409 ± 1.031	31.027	31.892
ENL	30.297 ± 0.511	30.058	30.735

5   Conclusion

In this paper, the US images of the knee joint cartilages of healthy subjects were evaluated. We attempted to remove the speckle noise, one of the downsides of US images while preserving the edges in US image. The AD method was used for this purpose and a scaled diffusivity function was proposed that preserves the edge and reduces the speckle noise in the output image. MAE is used as a stopping criterion between two consecutive diffusion iterations. Our numerical results show that the proposed method have substantially removed the speckle noise while preserve the edges efficiently.

Acknowledgement. This work was supported by Fundamental Research Grant Scheme (FRGS) FP092-2018A, Ministry of Education, Malaysia.

References

1. Jafarzadeh, S.R., Felson, D.T.: Updated estimates suggest a much higher prevalence of arthritis in United States adults than previous ones. Arthritis Rheumatol. **70**(2), 185–192 (2018)
2. Hossain, M.B., Lai, K.W., Pingguan-Murphy, B., Hum, Y.C., Mohd Salim, M.I., Liew, Y.M.: Contrast enhancement of ultrasound imaging of the knee joint cartilage for early detection of knee osteoarthritis. Biomed. Signal Process. Control **13**(1), 157–167 (2014)
3. Faisal, A., Ng, S.C., Goh, S.L., George, J., Supriyanto, E., Lai, K.W.: Multiple LREK active contours for knee meniscus ultrasound image segmentation. IEEE Trans. Med. Imaging **34**(10), 2162–2171 (2015)
4. Tur, M., Chin, K.C., Goodman, J.W.: When is speckle noise multiplicative? Appl. Opt. **21**(7), 1157 (1982)
5. Perona, P., Malik, J.: Scale-space and edge detection using anisotropic diffusion. IEEE Trans. Pattern Anal. Mach. Intell. **12**(7), 629–639 (1990)
6. Krissian, K., Westin, C.-F., Kikinis, R., Vosburgh, K.G.: Oriented speckle reducing anisotropic diffusion. IEEE Trans. Image Process. **16**(5), 1412–1424 (2007)
7. Zhang, F., Yoo, Y.M., Koh, L.M., Kim, Y.: Nonlinear diffusion in Laplacian pyramid domain for ultrasonic speckle reduction. IEEE Trans. Med. Imaging **26**(2), 200–211 (2007)
8. Ling, H., Bovik, A.C.: Smoothing low-SNR molecular images via anisotropic median-diffusion. IEEE Trans. Med. Imaging **21**(4), 377–384 (2002)
9. Kuan, D., Sawchuk, A., Strand, T., Chavel, P.: Adaptive restoration of images with speckle. IEEE Trans. Acoust. **35**(3), 373–383 (1987)
10. Aja-Fernandez, S., Alberola-Lopez, C.: On the estimation of the coefficient of variation for anisotropic diffusion speckle filtering. IEEE Trans. Image Process. **15**(9), 2694–2701 (2006)
11. Alvarez, L., Lions, P.-L., Morel, J.-M.: Image selective smoothing and edge detection by nonlinear diffusion. II. SIAM J. Numer. Anal. **29**(3), 845–866 (2005)
12. Yu, J., Tan, J., Wang, Y.: Ultrasound speckle reduction by a SUSAN-controlled anisotropic diffusion method. Pattern Recognit. **43**(9), 3083–3092 (2010)
13. Petrou, M., Petrou, C.: Image processing: the fundamentals (2010). https:\\www.it-ebooks. info
14. Black, M.J., Sapiro, G., Marimont, D.H., Heeger, D.: Robust anisotropic diffusion. IEEE Trans. Image Process. **7**(3), 421–432 (1998)
15. Hossain, M.B., Pingguan-Murphy, B., Chai Hum, Y., Wee Lai, K.: Contrast enhancement of ultrasound image of knee joint cartilage by using multipurpose beta optimized recursive bi-histogram equalization method, pp. 37–43 (2016)
16. Tsiotsios, C., Petrou, M.: On the choice of the parameters for anisotropic diffusion in image processing. Pattern Recognit. **46**(5), 1369–1381 (2013)
17. Wang, B., Chapron, B., Mercier, G., Garello, R., He, M.-X.: Polarimetric characteristics of ships on RADARSAT-2 data. In: OCEANS 2011 IEEE - Spain, pp. 1–4 (2011)

The Correlation of Model-Based Insulin Sensitivity and Respiratory P/F Score

A. Abu-Samah[1]([✉]), A. A. Razak[1], N. N. Razak[1], F. M. Suhaimi[2], and U. Jamaludin[3]

[1] Universiti Tenaga Nasional, 43000 Kajang, Malaysia
asma.abusamah@gmail.com
[2] Universiti Sains Malaysia, 13200 Bertam, Penang, Malaysia
[3] Universiti Malaysia Pahang, 26600 Pekan, Pahang, Malaysia

Abstract. Insulin resistance and impaired respiratory function have been associated together and have been suggested to be potential predictors for organ failures in ICU. Insulin resistance is however difficult to measure in real time especially in the case of critically-ill patients. ICING models enable the estimation of insulin sensitivity (SI) as a reflection of the resistance. Knowing their levels and of impaired lung function level could be useful first and foremost to determine potential respiratory organ failure. The relationship between them was studied using a retrospective data of 20 patients ((mean ± SD) age: 62.5 ± 12.2) admitted to the Universiti Malaya Medical Centre ICU, Kuala Lumpur. Data on gender, age, race, admission diagnosis and morbidities were collected in each patient. Correlation of per-patient SI to P/F (PO2/PiO2) score was determined using Pearson correlation score. In this single-centre study, results indicated that the generated SI can potentially replace insulin resistance measurement. Correlation scores were negatively high for 4 patients (< -8.0), but the data from respiratory side were small and unbalanced to generate any general pattern. In conclusion, the estimated SI can be used for further studies with more data to link and predict the decline of respiratory failure in the ICU.

Keywords: Insulin resistance · Insulin sensitivity · Lung failure · Respiratory failure · Organ failure

1 Introduction

Intensive care units (ICUs) treat critically-ill patients with multiple complications, and the common goal is the prevention of further organ dysfunction, the management of established organ failures and avoidance of mortality [1–3]. These patients with and without history of diabetes are however exposed to stress hyperglycaemia with associated mechanism such as insulin resistance, effect of medications and impaired glucose deficiency [4, 5]. In non-intensive care setting, several published studies suggested the association between reduced lung function, insulin resistance, Diabetes Mellitus, and cardiovascular disease development [6, 7]. Diabetes Mellitus is considered amongst the risk factors for the progress of obstructive lung disease [8]. The information on co-existence of impaired respiratory function, insulin resistance and Diabetes Mellitus has

© Springer Nature Switzerland AG 2021
F. Ibrahim et al. (Eds.): ICIBEL 2019, IFMBE Proceedings 81, pp. 54–62, 2021.
https://doi.org/10.1007/978-3-030-65092-6_6

been considered to improve treatment decision making as well as optimizing the clinical resources of both respiratory and glycaemic based failures [8]. In the same direction, current studies are initiated for ICU context.

Insulin resistance and glycaemic variation can be evaluated as a function of insulin sensitivity (SI) [9], a physiological parameter that describes the metabolic variation based on insulin concentration and glucose clearance. Insulin sensitivity is an inverse representation of insulin resistance. However in contrary to SI, there is no method yet to determine the resistance in real-time, and especially in the context of ICU [10]. ICING physiological model uses frequent available data such as blood glucose (BG) level, insulin deliverance and provided nutrition. It has the ability to estimate SI continuously. However based on current operation, input data are normally obtained hourly, thus allowing only hourly estimations of SI. ICING has been validated clinically and has been used extensively in different applications ranging from automated and personalized glycaemic control [11–15] to early detection of sepsis in ICU [16]. No prior study has been done on the association of the ICING-based insulin sensitivity and lung function health in critically-ill patients.

One of the most common score in the ICU used to diagnose the severity of lung function is the P/F ratio of partial pressure of oxygen PO2 (P) from the arterial blood gas test to the FiO2 (F), the fraction of inspired oxygen that a patient receives. The PO2 rises with increasing FiO2. Inadequate or decreased oxygen exchange decreases the ratio. It is one of the four criteria applied to define respiratory failure. The objective of the study is to determine if estimated insulin sensitivity using ICING model plays an associative role towards P/F score in patients admitted to Intensive Care Unit from Malaysia.

2   Methods

2.1   ICING Insulin Sensitivity Estimation

The model used to estimate SI is the clinically validated Intensive Care Insulin-Nutrition-Glucose (ICING) model. This model is built upon 7 equations which can be referred to in previous publications on SI model developments [17–19]. The equations describe the interaction between several physiological systems as shown in Fig. 1. Clinical inputs needed to compute each SI are; i) the BG level (in mmol/L); ii) administered insulin (in mU/L); and iii) provided nutrition to be translated into dextrose intake (in mmol/minute). Whilst the inputs are not provided every hour, SI (L.min/mU) can still be fitted hourly using integral-based fitting method [20]. SI estimation accuracy can be measured through BG fitting error. Each measured BG is compared with the estimated BG that produces hourly SI. ICING model SI estimation using integral-based fitting is guaranteed with less than 1% of fitting error.

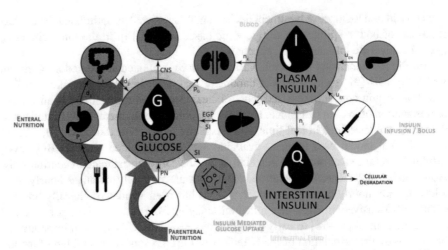

Fig. 1. The compartment representation of the physiological ICING model showing several functions; inputs and outputs linked to pancreas, intestine, stomach, central nervous system, liver and kidney [21].

2.2 Respiratory P/F Score

P/F score is commonly used measurement, in acute lung injury (ALI) and acute respiratory distress syndrome (ARDS) [22–24]. ALI describes the pulmonary response to a broad range of injuries occurring either directly to the lung or as a consequence of injury or inflammation at other sites of the body. ARDS represents the more severe end of this condition. P/F ratio of <300 defines ALI or mild ARDS, <200 to moderate ARDS and <100 alarms for severe ARDS. In the same way, the score is also adopted in Sequential Organ Failure Assessment (SOFA) [25] to track and to determine the extent of a person's organ function or rate of failure to six organs, including respiratory. The scores range from 0 to +4, going from fine to worst. A detection of change in daily SOFA score of ≥2 indicates that a patient is suffering from lung failure.

In the ICU, PO2 and FiO2 are measured and recorded separately according to clinical needs. For this study, P/F scores were collected whenever pO2 and FIO2 were available in the same record hour. Each patient's hourly SI was then compared with computed P/F score using Pearson correlation which measures the linear correlation between the two variables. It takes a range of values from +1 to −1. A value 0 quantifies no association between the two variables. A positive value indicates that as the value of one variable increases, so does the other, in positive association.

2.3 Patients Data and Correlation Study

20 patients' data were extracted for this study. Criteria of inclusion include, i) ICU stay between 24 h to 120 h and ii) Patients with minimal five P/F score. Patients detail can be referred to in Table 1. A total of 1297 h of SI estimations and 265 P/F scores were used in the study. 14 out of 20 patients were diagnosed with Diabetes Mellitus. Amongst the 14 patients, 11 patients had hypertension and 8 patients had dyslipidemia.

Table 1. Clinical details of all 20 patients.

Patient ID	Age	Sex	Race*	Admission condition	Comorbidity**	ICU stay (Day- hours)	Available P/F score	APACHE II Score
UM03	69	M	C	Post saucerization of right shoulder carbuncle with CAP	DM	3–67	16	8
UM09	64	M	M	Post drainage of ludwig's angina with severe metabolic acidosis, acute on CKD and sepsis	DM, HPT, Dyslipidemia, CKD	3–56	13	13
UM12	77	M	M	Post left nephrectomy for bosniak 3 renal cyst complicated by intraoperative presumed sepsis	DM, HPT, Dyslipidemia	2–33	6	24
UM19	44	M	M	Bilateral necrotizing pneumonia tro pulmonary tuberculosis	DM	5–108	22	23
UM20	48	M	C	OHF with CO2 narcosis, cover for pneumonia	OSA, CCF	2–39	10	10
UM23	39	M	M	Polytrauma with severe traumatic brain injury	None	4–74	15	17
UM29	74	F	C	Polytrauma secondary to motor vehicle accident	None	3–49	8	16
UM30	69	M	M	Septic shock secondary to right thigh abscess	DM, HPT, CKD	3–58	5	17
UM35	58	M	I	Atypical pneumonia with fluid overload, acute on CKD	DM, HPT, Dyslipidemia	5–110	22	20
UM37	68	F	C	Cardiogenic and septic shock (e.coli bacteremia)	DM, HPT, Ischaemic Heart Disease, End stage renal failure	4–74	6	27
UM43	78	M	C	Acute on chronic subdural hemorrhage with acute hydrocephalus, AKI and uncontrolled DM	DM, Dyslipidemia, Previous Ischaemic stroke	3–41	6	28
UM44	59	F	I	Dengue fever in critical phase with warning signs (lethargy, confusion, transaminitis)	DM, HPT, Dyslipidemia	4–87	29	11

(continued)

Table 1. (*continued*)

Patient ID	Age	Sex	Race*	Admission condition	Comorbidity**	ICU stay (Day- hours)	Available P/F score	APACHE II Score
UM45	71	F	M	Post exploratory laparotomy for caecal mass with intestinal obstruction	Severe primary hypothyroidism, Hypocortisolism	3–45	8	15
UM46	54	F	I	Dengue fever with transaminitis and uncontrolled DM	DM, HPT	4–93	44	14
UM48	69	F	I	Post right hemiglossectomy + right modified radical neck dissection, right hemithyroidectomy with right floor of mouth flap for right tongue squamous cell carcinoma	None	3–52	7	10
UM54	39	F	I	CAP	DM, HPT	4–87	17	17
UM56	73	F	M	Left lower limb necrotizing fasciitis post wound debridement and fasciotomy	DM, HPT, Dyslipidemia	4–57	7	7
UM58	73	F	M	Post laparotomy for obstructed splenic flexure tumour with bowel ischaemia complicated with metabolic acidosis	None	4–65	9	
UM60	64	M	M	Sepsis secondary to infected diabetic foot ulcer with severe metabolic acidosis and hyperlactataemia	DM, HPT, Dyslipidemia, IHD	2–35	10	
UM61	60	M	C	Recurrent stroke, cover for pneumonia	DM, HPT, Dyslipidemia, stroke	3–67	5	

*M: Malay, I: Indian and C: Chinese
**AKI: Acute Kidney Injury, DM: Diabetes Mellitus, CAP: Community Acquired Pneumonia, CCF: Congestive Cardiac Failure, CKD: Chronic Kidney Disease, HPT: Hypertension, IHD: Ischemic Heart Disease, and OSA: Obstructive Sleep Apnea,

3 Results

Figure 2 shows the scatter plot of all 167 estimated SI values with associated P/F scores. The majority of patients with existing P/F score had lower than 0.001 mmol/min SI. This group's median and IQR SI are 15.16 [4.43–39.09]10^{-5} L.min/mU. Low SI indicates higher insulin resistance, found in this cohort. In particular, 236 had zero SI which indicated SI in the order of 10^{-7}. The percentage of P/F score in each range; <100 to >400 are displayed on the right hand of the graph, highlighting a slightly skewed distribution towards better respiratory condition of patients.

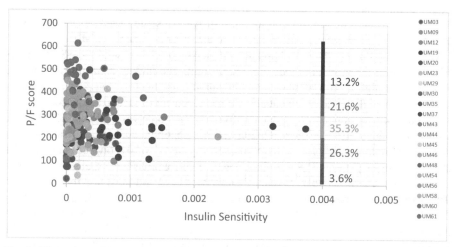

Fig. 2. The scatter plot of insulin sensitivity vs. P/F score. The P/F score distribution (%) can be referred to on the right side of the graph.

Figure 3 illustrates the correlation score between SI and P/F score for all patients. The graph distinguishes the diabetic from the non-diabetic patients using red bars. According to this, 11 have negative values. Most had more than −0.2 correlation, and patient UM30 had a perfect negative correlation. Those with positive values have lower than +0.4 correlation.

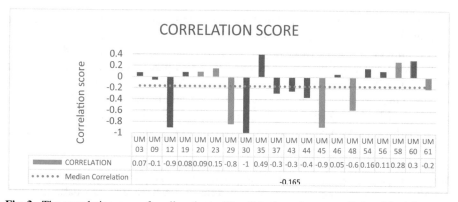

Fig. 3. The correlation score for all patients. The diabetic patients are distinguished from the non-diabetics using red bars.

4 Discussion

Our findings revealed that in particular, at times where PO2 and FiO2 record existed in the same hour, the associated estimated SI were very low, indicating the existence of high insulin resistance for most of studied patients. The median SI was 15.16 [4.43–39.09] 10^{-5} L.min/mU. In this cohort, 3.6% of the P/F scores were below 100, which is the lower limit of severe ARDS and were affecting 3 patients (UM03, UM23 and UM35). These three patients had positive P/F score correlation with their SI variation. 61.6% were in the mild and moderate ARDS limit. The finding confirms not only the link between high insulin resistance and impaired lung function, but also the usability of the estimated SIs to complement clinical measurement of insulin resistance.

Some patients showed very high negative correlation between SI and the P/F score whilst many stays within ±0.4 correlation which is important but not significant. Studies on their demographic, admission diagnosis, severity APACHE II score and comorbidities showed no clear pattern. The 4 highest negative correlations nevertheless share some common characteristics such as older than 69 years old and have less than 60 h stay. The pattern either doesn't exist, or it could be attributed to the low ratio of available SI over P/F scores (1297:265). We believe better correlation scores can be obtained if we interpolate the P/F score to match the number of hourly SI. With the availability of the interpolated data, more studies on time series development can equally be performed.

Two studies using limited and irregular data showed a close association between Diabetes Mellitus and hypertension towards estimated SI-based glycaemic control results, using Bayesian Network [26, 27]. Bayesian Network is an approach that use correlation weight to develop probabilistical causal or risk models. Another perspective from these studies is to use Bayesian Network to model the co-relationship between the various elements existing in current data.

5 Conclusion

Insulin resistance should be considered amongst the risk factors for deterioration in lung function. However, their usage is clinically limited in decision making as the measurement is difficult to obtain, especially in the ICU. This suggests exploring the usage of model-based generated insulin sensitivity which is a parameter that is the inverse of insulin resistance. Current intention however must be supported with more generated data from the respiratory side. Subsequent studies with bigger and sufficient data will include the SI role to predict lung failure in advance based on time series model. SI-based prediction may lead to effective interventions targeting respective organ failure prevention.

Acknowledgment. The authors thankfully acknowledge Universiti Malaya Medical Centre (UMMC) ICU clinical team, specifically Dr. Tan Ru Yi, Dr. Khaironisa Abu Bakar and Prof. Mohamad Shahnaz Hassan for their support and this study's data provision. The authors also acknowledge FRGS Grant FRGS/1/2019/STG05/UNITEN/02/1 from the Malaysian Ministry of Education MOE and BOLD+UNIIG grant from UNITEN for their parts in the current research.

References

1. Yamada, T., Shojima, N., Noma, H., Yamauchi, T., Kadowaki, T.: Glycemic control, mortality, and hypoglycemia in critically ill patients: a systematic review and network meta-analysis of randomized controlled trials. Intensiv. Care Med. **43**(1), 1–15 (2017)
2. Oz, E., Salturk, C., Karakurt, Z., Yazicioglu Mocin, O., Adiguzel, N., Gungor, G., Devran, O., Kalamanoglu, M., Horzum, G., Yilmaz, A.: Risk factors for multi-organ failure and mortality in severe sepsis patients who need intensive care unit follow-up. Tuberkuloz ve toraks **63**(3), 147–157 (2015)
3. Krinsley, J.S.: Association between hyperglycemia and increased hospital mortality in a heterogeneous population of critically ill patients. In: Mayo Clinic Proceedings, vol. 78, no. 12, pp. 1471–1478. Elsevier (December 2003)
4. Dungan, K.M., Braithwaite, S.S., Preiser, J.C.: Stress hyperglycaemia. Lancet **373**, 1798–1807 (2009)
5. McCowen, K.C., Malhotra, A., Bistrian, B.R.: Stress-induced hyperglycemia. Crit. Care Clin. **17**(1), 107–124 (2001)
6. Sagun, G., Gedik, C., Ekiz, E., Karagoz, E., Takir, M., Oguz, A.: The relation between insulin resistance and lung function: a cross sectional study. BMC Pulm. Med. **15**(1), 139 (2015)
7. Ormazabal, V., Nair, S., Elfeky, O., Aguayo, C., Salomon, C., Zuñiga, F.A.: Association between insulin resistance and the development of cardiovascular disease. Cardiovasc. Diabetol. **17**(1), 122 (2018)
8. Mirrakhimov, A.E.: Chronic obstructive pulmonary disease and glucose metabolism: a bitter sweet symphony. Cardiovasc. Diabetol. **11**(1), 132 (2012)
9. Chase, J.G., Le Compte, A.J., Suhaimi, F., Shaw, G.M., Lynn, A., Lin, J., Pretty, C.G., Razak, N., Parente, J.D., Hann, C.E., Preiser, J.C.: Tight glycemic control in critical care–the leading role of insulin sensitivity and patient variability: a review and model-based analysis. Comput. Methods Programs Biomed. **102**(2), 156–171 (2012)
10. Borai, A., Livingstone, C., Kaddam, I., Ferns, G.: Selection of the appropriate method for the assessment of insulin resistance. BMC Med. Res. Methodol. **11**(1), 158 (2011)
11. Evans, A., Le Compte, A., Tan, C.S., Ward, L., Steel, J., Pretty, C.G., Chase, J.G.: Stochastic targeted (STAR) glycemic control: design, safety, and performance. J. Diabetes Sci. Technol. **6**(1), 102–115 (2012)
12. Penning, S., Le Compte, A.J., Moorhead, K.T., Desaive, T., Massion, P., Preiser, J.C., Chase, J.G.: First pilot trial of the STAR-Liege protocol for tight glycemic control in critically ill patients. Comput. Methods Programs Biomed. **108**(2), 844–859 (2012)
13. Blaha, J., Barteczko-Grajek, B., Berezowicz, P., Charvat, J., Chvojka, J., Grau, T., Starkopf, J.: Space glucose control system for blood glucose control in intensive care patients - a European multicentre observational study. BMC Anesthesiol. **16**(1), 8 (2016)
14. Abu-Samah, A., Dickson, J.L., Abdul Razak, N.N., Abdul Razak, A., Jamaludin, U.K., Mohamad Suhaimi, F., Pretty, C.G.: Model-based glycemic control in a Malaysian intensive care unit: performance and safety study. Med. Devices: Evid. Res. **12**, 215–226 (2019)
15. Chase, J.G., Benyo, B., Desaive, T.: Glycemic control in the intensive care unit: a control systems perspective. Ann. Rev. Control **48**, 359–368 (2019)
16. Suhaimi, F.M., Jamaludin, U.K., Razak, N.N., Pretty, C.G., Ralib, A.M., Nor, M.B., Dzaharudin, F.: Blood glucose and sepsis score on sepsis patients requiring insulin therapy. In: International Conference for Innovation in Biomedical Engineering and Life Sciences, pp. 265–269 (December 2017)
17. Lin, J., Razak, N.N., Pretty, C.G., Le Compte, A., Docherty, P., Parente, J.D., Shaw, G.M., Hann, C.E., Chase, J.G.: A physiological intensive control insulin-nutrition-glucose (ICING) model validated in critically ill patients. Comput. Methods Programs Biomed. **102**(2), 192–205 (2011)

18. Pretty, C.G., Le Compte, A., Penning, S., Fisk, L., Shaw, G.M., Desaive, T., Chase, J.G.: Interstitial insulin kinetic parameters for a 2-compartment insulin model with saturable clearance. Comput. Methods Programs Biomed. **114**(3), e39–e45 (2014)
19. Stewart, K.W., Pretty, C.G., Tomlinson, H., Fisk, L., Shaw, G.M., Chase, J.G.: Stochastic model predictive (stomp) glycaemic control for the intensive care unit: development and virtual trial validation. Biomed. Signal Process. Control **16**, 61–67 (2015)
20. Hann, C.E., Chase, J.G., Lin, J., Lotz, T., Doran, C.V., Shaw, G.M.: Integral-based parameter identification for long-term dynamic verification of a glucose–insulin system model. Comput. Methods Programs Biomed. **77**(3), 259–270 (2005)
21. Uyttendaele, V., Dickson, J.L., Shaw, G.M., Desaive, T., Chase, J.G.: Untangling glycaemia and mortality in critical care. Crit. Care **21**(1), 152 (2017)
22. Irish Critical Care Trials Group: Acute lung injury and the acute respiratory distress syndrome in Ireland: a prospective audit of epidemiology and management. Crit. Care **12**(1), R30 (2008)
23. Singh, G., Gladdy, G., Chandy, T.T., Sen, N.: Incidence and outcome of acute lung injury and acute respiratory distress syndrome in the surgical intensive care unit. Indian J. Crit. Care Med.: Peer-Rev. Off. Publ. Indian Soc. Crit. Care Med. **18**(10), 659 (2014)
24. Griffiths, M.J., McAuley, D.F., Perkins, G.D., Barrett, N., Blackwood, B., Boyle, A., Chee, N., Connolly, B., Dark, P., Finney, S., Salam, A.: Guidelines on the management of acute respiratory distress syndrome. BMJ Open Respir. Res. **6**(1), e000420 (2019)
25. Vincent, J.L., Moreno, R., Takala, J., Willatts, S., De Mendonca, A., Bruining, H., Reinhart, C.K., Suter, P., Thijs, L.G.: The SOFA (sepsis-related organ failure assessment) score to describe organ dysfunction/failure. On behalf of the working group on sepsis-related problems of the European society of intensive care medicine. Intensiv. Care Med. **22**, 707–710 (1996)
26. Abu-Samah, A., Razak, N.N., Suhaimi, F.M., Jamaludin, U.K., Chase, G.: Linking Bayesian network and intensive care units data: a glycemic control study. In: TENCON 2018-2018 IEEE Region 10 Conference, pp. 1988–1993. IEEE (October 2018)
27. Abu-Samah, A., Razak, N.N., Suhaimi, F.M., Jamaludin, U.K., Ralib, A.M.: Probabilistic glycemic control decision support in ICU: proof of concept using bayesian network. Jurnal Teknologi **81**(2), 61–69 (2019)

Tracking of Near-Field Wireless Transceiver for Implantable Devices

Teh Chong Cheng[1], Mohd Yazed Bin Ahmad[2], and Noraisyah Mohamed Shah[1](✉)

[1] Department of Electrical Engineering, Faculty of Engineering, University of Malaya,
50603 Kuala Lumpur, Malaysia
noraisyah@um.edu.my
[2] Department of Biomedical Engineering, Faculty of Engineering, University of Malaya,
50603 Kuala Lumpur, Malaysia
myaz@um.edu.my

Abstract. Wireless Capsule Endoscopy (WCE) is used in wireless near-field transceiver system to achieve localization aim along with a loop antenna as main transmitter coil used for power transmission while receiving localization data. The receiving antenna is installed in WCE to receive power and as coupling antenna. Both antennas are matched to ensure maximum power transfer through 5MHz electromagnetic wave. FEKO simulation software was used to complete the initial stage design and data acquisition. Multiple simulations were completed in all coordinates in the transmitter coil antenna region. Using MATLAB curve fitting toolbox on to the collected data, a suitable polynomial was considered to design the localization algorithm. The proposed polynomial equation to fit the actual data had gained over 90% of accuracy and the model was able to achieve localization in a circular locus.

Keywords: Wireless capsule endoscopy · Localization · Coil antenna · Near-field wireless transceiver

1 Introduction

1.1 Overview

Internal disease such as internal bleeding, ulcer or tumor that existed in the gastrointestinal tract (GI tract) when not handled well during the early stages may turn up into serious illnesses [1]. Yet, the use of various diagnostics methods such as X-ray, or other types of traditional endoscopy alternatives were not as effective as WCE when opting for a less invasive solution [2]. It was reported that the above methodologies had returned a non-impactful result as the diagnostics yield were low even when used in the detection of an internal bleeding [3]. A camera that is attached on capsule's head is used to record and capture internal images can be used effectively in determining internal bleeding of the gastrointestinal tract. This wireless capsule is of a swallowable size, with dimensions equivalent to a large vitamin pill, about 25 mm [4].

© Springer Nature Switzerland AG 2021
F. Ibrahim et al. (Eds.): ICIBEL 2019, IFMBE Proceedings 81, pp. 63–67, 2021.
https://doi.org/10.1007/978-3-030-65092-6_7

2 Research Methodology

2.1 Process Flow

The HF frequency range (3–30 MHz) is the frequency range adopted. The loop antenna is selected as it has a very small radiation resistance property for electrically-small application that are widely used in near-field application [5]. As the receiver coil's position is varied along a constant axis, the value of the impedance of the system was acquired and analysed for localization purpose. Using the FEKO simulation software, the receiver coil is placed at different position along the z-axis first to acquire the impedance data of the simulation. The initial solution for positioning the z-axis was proposed after considering all factors (Fig. 1).

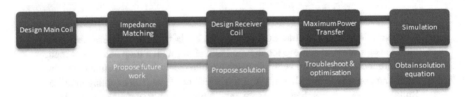

Fig. 1. Main process flow of the whole project

2.2 Main Transmitter Coil and Receiver Coil

The coil antenna structure was sketched using the CADFEKO software. A current carrying loop was first designed and the parameters were initially set to simulate a simple coil structure. The parameters set were as below:

1. Frequency: 5 MHz
2. Number of Turns, N = 5
3. Voltage Source = 12 V
4. Copper Wire Cross-section diameter = 0.15 cm (~AWG15 copper wire)

For electrically-small antennas, the overall length of circumference (C) is near to or less than one tenth of the actual wavelength. (C < λ/10) [6]. Since speed of light, $c = f\lambda$. If we let $\lambda = 10\lambda$, then $10\lambda = c/f$, with f = 5 MHz, we obtained $\lambda = 600$ cm.

The receiver coil is being designed to fit into the pill-sized capsule. The parameters are set as below:

1. Radius: 0.6 cm
2. Number of Turns, N = 10
3. Copper Wire Cross-section diameter = 0.45 mm

2.3 Data Acquisition

To acquire the impedance of the main transmitter (Tx) coil due to changes of location in receiver (Rx) coil, a parameter sweep needs to be performed using simulation. The height is manipulated by altering the value in the variable that is assigned to the translation axis. The receiver position is resolved into a Cartesian coordinate system where xyz axis are used to represent the receiver's position. As the radius of the receiver coil is 0.6 cm, the parametric sweep is set a few limits from radius of 0 cm to 16 cm and height is set from 0 cm to 20 cm. The antenna is first designed as a three-coil loop antenna, with upper and lower region separated by a middle coil antenna.

2.4 Localization Algorithm

The acquired impedance simulation data in real and imaginary components, was transferred into Microsoft Excel for further analysis. The Real and Imaginary value varies with the changes in position of the receiver coil. A conditional formatting is applied to the data to find any duplicated values to check for possible ambiguous cases where the values is similar at two different position. In MATLAB, the data is plotted in 3D using the polynomial linear model of the curve fitting toolbox. The optimum result was achieved by changing the degree of each variable to reduce the complexity of the polynomial equation and thus achieving the optimum goodness of fit of the data with the equation. Judging from the curve fitting accuracy, R-squared, the Polynomial equation degree is then adjusted to reduce the complexity of the whole equation. Since the degree of the polynomial equation is the same for both part of the impedances, the base equation is the same, as given in Eq. (1) below. The coefficients are then substituted into the base equation to obtain the final characteristic equation for both real part and imaginary part, z1_real, z1_img, z2_real, z2_img.

$$
\begin{aligned}
f(x, y) = &\, p00 + p10x + p01y + p20x2 + p11xy + p02y^2 + p30x^3 + p21x^2y \\
&+ p12xy^2 + p03y^3 + p40x^4 + p31x^3y + p22x^2y^2 + p13xy^3 + p04y^4 \\
&+ p50x^5 + p41x^4y + p32x^3y^2 + p23x^2y^3 + p14xy^4
\end{aligned}
\tag{1}
$$

The proposed solution to acquire the position is given in the flowchart of Fig. 2.

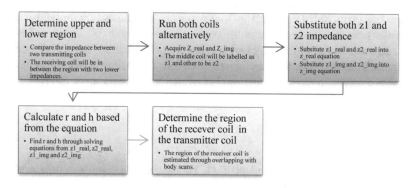

Fig. 2. Flowchart of the localization algorithm

3   Result and Discussion

The current project managed to achieve a circle locus which greatly narrows down the area of the receiver coil to a circular path. The result returns more than 90% goodness of fit of data (R-squared > 0.9).

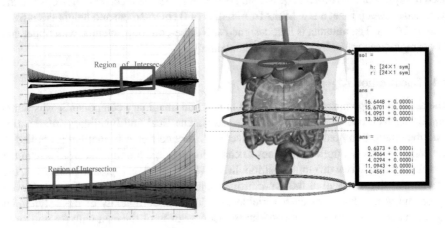

Fig. 3.   Result of test run

Figure 3 explains the region of the receiver coil is estimated by overlapping through a sample scan of human body with the coordinates plotted from the results. The result is to be determined by comparing with the body scan of GI tract.

4   Conclusion and Future Work

Considering that the polynomial equation returns multiple roots, these roots need to be filtered according to the region of interest. The accuracy of the solution will vary due to the inconsistent number of roots within the region of interest.

To achieve a more precise region, the introduction of secondary coil structure (auxiliary coil) can be included in the design to provide another dimension for intersection of the circular path that further reduces the region of the receiver coil. Besides, few algorithms had been also discovered including using comparison of mathematical modeling, using artificial intelligence such as linear regression. It is believed that the behavior of impedance changes in the transmitter coil is related to the function of the H-field for a coil loop antenna.

References

1. Caffrey, C.M., Chevalerias, O., Mathuna, C.O., Twomey, K.: Swallowable-capsule technology. IEEE Pervasive Comput. **7**(1), 23–29 (2008)

2. Wang, Y., Ding, N., Wu, X., Li, D., Yu, J.: Averaging position algorithm of an independent rotating coils based electromagnetic tracking system (2013)
3. Lewis, B.S.: Small intestinal bleeding. Gastroenterol Clin North Am **29**(1), 67–95 (2000). (in eng), K. Elissa
4. Britannica, T.E.O.E.: Magnetic dipole, June 08, 2017, November. https://www.britannica.com/science/magnetic-dipole
5. Balanis, C.A.J.P.O.T.I.: Antenna theory: a review. Proc. IEEE **80**(1), 7–23 (1992)
6. Bevelacqua, P.J.: Small Loop Antennas, Loop Antennas

Modelling of Transcranial Magnetic Stimulation (TMS) Induced Fields in Different Age Groups

Mansour Alawi[1], Lee Poh Foong[1(✉)], Goh Yong Kheng[1], Deng Zhi-De[2], and Paul E. Croarkin[3]

[1] Lee Kong Chien Faculty of Engineering and Sciences, Universiti Tunku Abdul Rahman, Petaling Jaya, Selangor, Malaysia
leepf@utar.edu.my
[2] Noninvasive Neuromodulation Unit, National Institute of Mental Health, NIH, Bethesda, USA
[3] Department of Psychiatry and Psychology, Mayo Clinic, Rochester, MN, USA

Abstract. Transcranial magnetic stimulation (TMS) is non-invasive brain stimulation procedure adopting the intense magnetic pulses to induce an electric field in neuronal tissue, modulating cortical excitability level. Computational modelling and simulation have played a major role in the development of many TMS therapeutic applications for adults such as Major Depression Disorder (MDD) treatment. However, TMS is still being investigated in pediatric and geriatric for numerous clinical applications and conditions due to physiological differences from adults. Studies of TMS induced fields' effect comparison were usually limited to two age groups Child/Adult or Adult/Elderly, our study included a comparison of three widely spread age groups Child, Adult and Elderly. This study aimed to simulate the strength and distribution of TMS induced electric fields in an MRI base head model of different age groups. Child, Adult and Elderly head MRI images were used. Individualized finite-element method modelling of the TMS induced electric field at the head vertex (Cz) was performed. The profound outcome from the work displays a notable higher TMS induced electric field and larger field expansion in the Grey and White matters of Child and Elderly samples in compare to Adult. The head model for these three groups shows an obvious difference in the white and grey matters of the brain composition. The underdevelopment brain size for children, and shrinking of brain composition for elderlies are very similar. This important point has explained the electric field strength on the brain. The usefulness of the TMS modelling effects on the brain for different age groups may serve patients better for a wider age range.

Keywords: TMS · Simulation · Modelling · Age groups · Induced electric field

1 Introduction

Transcranial magnetic stimulation (TMS) is a noninvasive tool that uses electromagnetic induction principles to stimulate and modulate the neural activities in certain targeted areas in the brain [1]. Pulses from TMS are brief and intense magnetic pulses are generated by passing a high electric current through an electromagnetic coil placed above

© Springer Nature Switzerland AG 2021
F. Ibrahim et al. (Eds.): ICIBEL 2019, IFMBE Proceedings 81, pp. 68–75, 2021.
https://doi.org/10.1007/978-3-030-65092-6_8

the scalp, such magnetic pulse can induce electric fields and intracerebral currents in the brain that depolarize neurons and alter cortical functions [2]. From the first introduction of this method more than 3-decade ago, TMS has turned into an important therapeutic and diagnostic tool in the neurology, neurophysiology, neurosurgery and psychiatry fields, together with its usage for the studying of cortex functional mapping [3]. The application of TMS on adults are wide which it serves as a tool to diagnose [4] and treat different types of neurological and psychiatric disorders such as stroke, epilepsy and depression. The preliminary success of this technique for the adults have promoted for a similar beneficial development for pediatric and geriatric settings [5].

The usage of TMS in children and the elderly population is just emerging and facing many limitations and challenges related to the maturation and degradation of the brain behaviourally and neurophysiologically [6]. Identifying the effects of the brain size and brain tissue anatomical differences along the life-span on the TMS treatment are believed to play a role in more precise quantification of dosing [3]. Few studies only have addressed the variability of the TMS-induced fields in the Adult\Child, Adult\Elderly brain models [3, 7]. Most of those simulation outcomes were impressive in distinguishing the age effects on TMS induced fields. However, the lack of age-dependent parameters along life-span and the usage of spherical or smoothed brain surface head models, have risen then need to conduct a comparison study that uses realistic head model to compare TMS induced fields in Child\Adult\Elderly altogether.

In this study, we aim to report the simulation effect of the distribution and electric field strength of the TMS on subjects that consisted of three different ages and stages of human life with their 3D realistic head models generated from high-resolution MRI images. This may potentially provide a predictive dosage of TMS treatment and its effects on these three different age groups and hence increasing the efficiency and safety for the treatment.

2 Methodology

2.1 Sample Recruitment

(See Table 1).

Table 1. Selected sample group and the ages categories

Group	Sample age (years old)
Child [8]	8
Adult [9]	30
Elderly [10]	75

2.2 TMS Fields' Simulation

Transcranial magnetic stimulation electric field modelling was performed using the SimNIBS pipeline version 2.1.2 [11]. Briefly, The MRI images were reoriented into Radiological (LAS) coordination, and voxel size standardised to [1 1 1] to allow easier result comparison. The anatomical volumes of each sample T1 MRI images were segmented into five types of tissues using MATLAB (Mathworks, MA), SPM12 [12] and CAT12. Via the SIMNIBS headreco function. The five segmentation surfaces are corresponding to Skin, Skull, Cerebrospinal fluid (CSF), Grey Matter (GM), and White Matter (WM). The segmentations were visually examined slice-by-slice to ensure accuracy and proper tissue classifications with Freeview [13]. Consequently, the tetrahedral volumes mesh 3D head models were created based on the segmentation surfaces using SimNIBS, mesh and simulated electric field were visualized using Gmsh [14]. Table 2 shows the conductivity values for each tissue type were used in FEM calculation [15].

Table 2. Head tissues conductivity values

Tissue type	Conductivity value Siemens/meter (S/m)
'WM'	0.126
'GM'	0.275
'CSF'	1.654
'Bone'	0.01
'Scalp'	0.465

2.3 Simulation Coil Placement

SimNIBS' virtual TMS Figure-of-Eight Magstim 70-mm coil was used ON the generated 3D head models as shown in Fig. 1. The coil positioning was conforming according to the EEG 10-10 electrodes positions [16], that created individually based on each head model anatomical characteristics. The coil centre was placed on the model Cz position (Head vertex) in this study, the coil Y-axis were parallel and in the same direction of 3D head models anterior–posterior orientation. The coil centre was set to be at 2 mm (mm) above the scalp to take into account the hair thickness.

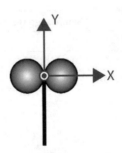

Fig. 1. Simulation coil Figure-of-Eight (Fo8) directions' reference.

2.4 Field Modelling

In the Visual Modelling, by using the similar coil current strength on all head model (strength B) Table 3, two views for the electric field were considered. Firstly a transverse plane view to show the spread of the electric field on the cortex (Top view), meanwhile the second view was on a coronal cutting plane at the center of the coil to show the propagation of the electric field induced into the grey and white matter (front view). The Numerical Modelling has been done base on collecting and comparing the peaks of the electric field induced by TMS in both brain grey and white matters under three different coil current strengths Table 3. However, to avoid outlier effects, the peak values were defined as the 99.9th percentile after arranging the electric field values in each tissue in ascending order.

Table 3. The Figure-of-eight coil currents used in the modelling the effects of the TMS induced electric field

Modelling type	Coil current strength Ampere/second		
	Strength A	Strength B	Strength C
	100[a]	150[a]	200[a]
Visual		✓	
Numerical	✓	✓	✓

[a] $\times 10^4$ Ampere/second (A/s)

3 Results

3.1 Field Visualization

After running the simulation with SimNIBS on the three 3D head models using the parameters listed in Table 2 and Coil current (strength B) Table 3, a visualizations for the simulated electric field using different views were generated. The fields' distribution on the cortex using a transverse plane view on the top of the head models is shown in Fig. 2(A), whereas the field distribution in the brain's gray and white matters was shown Fig. 2(B) by using a coronal plane view that cut the head model on the coil center of the simulation.

The visual brain map is displayed in Fig. 2(A) and 2(B), the figures show an obvious result for the same simulation parameters, the Child and Elderly population were experiencing a higher values in terms of the generated electric field in comparison to Adult population.

In Fig. 2(B), the images of the GM and WM shows that the TMS induced electric field difference was not only on the cortex surface Fig. 2(A), but the difference was also in terms of the field expansion into the brain tissues. The coronal cutting plane used in Fig. 2(B) has shown the field depth into the brain tissues, the TMS induced electric field depth were higher in Child and Elderly in compare to Adult similar to the effect seen on the cortex. Besides that, electric field strengths were seen to be higher in the gray matter in comparison to the white matter which is deeper and further from the coil.

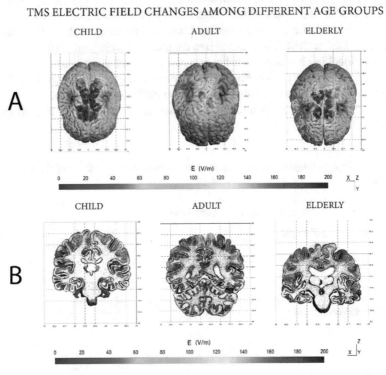

Fig. 2. Visual Modelling of the TMS induced electric fields in the brain of different age groups (A) Transverse plane view (Top view), the highest electric field strength can be seen in child's brain in compare to elderly which is higher than adult (B) Coronal cutting plane (front view), higher electric field propagation in GM and WM of the child, adult and elderly.

3.2 Simulation Strength Effect

In Fig. 3, display for the effects of the different coil currents on the peak of TMS induced electric field were shown. Three different current strengths were applied over all the 3D head models. The peak value for each field were compared among the different age groups and brain tissue. In all the 3D head models, the field's peak value has shown a direct proportional relation to the simulation coil's current strengths. In other words, for the same 3D head model the lowest peak was associated with the lowest current strength and vice versa.

An overview for peaks of the TMS induced electric field in WM and GM under all different coil currents has given the least peak values to the tissues of Adult group in compare to Child and Elderly groups. Whereas, the TMS induced electric field peaks in WM and GM were the highest in Child Group. Elderly group have shown an in-between peaks value in comparing to Child and Adult groups. However, it can be seen that the peak difference between the Child\Elderly groups is significantly smaller to the peak difference between Child\Adults and Elderly\Adults. Under the same coil current the WM of all groups have shown a significantly lower TMS induced electric field peak in compare to the GM of the same group.

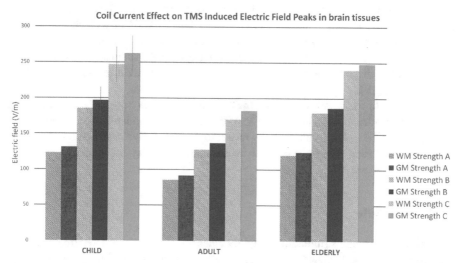

Fig. 3. Shows the simulated electric field peaks resulted from different coil current strengths (Red: coil current 1, Blue: coil Current 2, Green: Coil current 3) in different brain tissues (faded color: WM, Solid color: GM) of different age groups. TMS induced electric field was the highest in Child then Elderly end with Adult under all coil currents. Besides that, the induced electric field in the GM was higher than the induced electric field in WM in all groups and under all coil currents. Finally, the highest coil current have shown the highest electric field peak and vice versa.

4 Discussion

In this study, we modelled TMS induced electric fields with 3D head models generated from MRI anatomy of individual form different age groups, consisted of Child, Adult and Elderly. The result has demonstrated that the children may experience a stronger and more widespread electric field on their head for TMS simulation in compare to elderly and adults. Furthermore, the simulated results from elderly are shown equally high in the effected electric field peak as compared to the adults. This might due to the age-related differences such as the skull size besides the physiology developmental changes occurring through the human life-span in the grey and white matters. Individualized electric field modelling may play a big role in personalizing the effective dosage of TMS in future for both pediatrics and geriatric treatment and clinical trials.

To the best of our knowledge, this is the only study that model the TMS induced fields in samples age varying from Child to Adult and Elderly. We found significantly the highest peak of TMS induced electric field, and the most expansive electric field spread for children compared to Adult and elderly. These findings may relate to thinner skulls of children associated with head anatomical development compared to adults. Skull is much less conductive than other tissue and therefore reduces the transmission of the electric field generated by TMS [15], our results suggest that thinner skulls of children may reduce electric field blockage, resulting in a more electric field is reaching the inner tissues i.e. GM, WM. The TMS induced electric field in the Elderly have shown a higher peak value in comparison to adults. Such a difference might be linked to the skull thinning associated with aging [17]. On the other hand, the Elderly electric field peak was observed to be trivially lower than the Child that can be reasoned to the shrinking in the brain volume which increases the distance between the scalp and the cortex, such increase in the distance reduces the strength of the electric field reaching the Elderly GM and WM [18].

The effect of the distance between the coil and tissue can be seen when comparing the induced electric field in GM and WM of the same group under the same coil current strength. The GM which is anatomically nearer to the coil always shown a higher induced field than WM, such difference can also be reasoned to the tissue conductivity which is in favour of the GM.

5   Conclusion

Transcranial magnetic stimulation is rapidly emerging as a diagnosis and treatment tool for different illnesses. However, the head anatomical difference during humans' life-span can affect the efficacy of TMS treatment. Therefore, simulation and modelling of the TMS induced electric field on different age groups were carried out. Overall, the inducing electric field shows the highest peak in Child group, which proceeded by Elderly group and the lowest field peaks was on the Adult group. Direct proportional relation between the coil current and the induced electric field were demonstrated as well. Further work can be done in the future to prove the TMS induced electric field effects on larger sample groups from different ages.

References

1. Barker, A.T., Jalinous, R., Freeston, I.L.: Non-invasive magnetic stimulation of human motor cortex. Lancet1(8437), 1106–1107 (1985). https://linkinghub.elsevier.com/retrieve/pii/S01 40673685924134
2. Cvetković, M., Poljak, D., Rogić Vidaković, M., Đogaš, Z.: Transcranial magnetic stimulation induced fields in different brain models. J. Electromagn. Waves Appl. 30(14), 1820–1835 (2016)
3. Fischl, B., et al.: Automatically parcellating the human cerebral cortex. Cereb. Cortex 14(1), 11–22 (2004)
4. Frye, R.E., Rotenberg, A., Ousley, M., Pascual-Leone, A.: Transcranial magnetic stimulation in child neurology: current and future directions. J. Child Neurol. 23(1), 79–96 (2008)
5. George, M.S., et al.: Daily left prefrontal transcranial magnetic stimulation therapy for major depressive disorder. Arch. Gen. Psychiatry67(5), 507 (2010). https://archpsyc.jamanetwork. com/article.aspx?doi=10.1001/archgenpsychiatry.2010.46

6. Geuzaine, C., Remacle, J.-F.: Gmsh: a 3-D finite element mesh generator with built-in pre- and post-processing facilities. Int. J. Numer. Methods Eng. **79**(11), 1309–1331 (2009). https://doi.org/10.1002/nme.2579

7. Jurcak, V., Tsuzuki, D., Dan, I.: 10/20, 10/10, and 10/5 systems revisited: their validity as relative head-surface-based positioning systems. NeuroImage **34**(4), 1600–1611 (2007)

8. Lee, E.G., et al.: Investigational effect of brain-scalp distance on the efficacy of transcranial magnetic stimulation treatment in depression. IEEE Trans. Magn. **52**(7), 10–13 (2016)

9. Lepping, R.J., Atchley, R.A., Savage, C.R.: Development of a validated emotionally provocative musical stimulus set for research. Psychol. Music **44**(5), 1012–1028 (2016). https://doi.org/10.1177/0305735615604509. This data was obtained from the OpenNeuro database. Its accession number is ds000171

10. Lillie, E.M., et al.: Evaluation of skull cortical thickness changes with age and sex from computed tomography scans. J. Bone Miner. Res. **31**(2), 299–307 (2016)

11. Lu, M., Ueno, S.: A comparison of induced electric fields in child and adult head models by transcranial magnetic stimulation. In: 2011 XXXth General Assembly and Scientific Symposium, URSI, vol. 1, no. c, pp. 1–4 (2011)

12. Opitz, A., et al.: Determinants of the electric field during transcranial direct current stimulation. NeuroImage **109**, 140–150 (2015). https://doi.org/10.1016/j.neuroimage.2015.01.033

13. Penny, W., et al.: Statistical parametric mapping: the analysis of functional brain images (2007)

14. Petrov, P.I., et al.: How much detail is needed in modeling a transcranial magnetic stimulation figure-8 coil: measurements and brain simulations. PLoS ONE **12**(6), 1–20 (2017)

15. Rajapakse, T., Kirton, A.: Non-invasive brain stimulation in children: applications and future directions. Transl. Neurosci.**4**(2), 217–233 (2013). https://www.degruyter.com/view/j/tnsci.2013.4.issue-2/s13380-013-0116-3/s13380-013-0116-3.xml

16. Richardson, H., Lisandrelli, G., Riobueno-Naylor, A., Saxe, R.: Development of the social brain from age three to twelve years. Nat. Commun. **9**(1), 1027 (2018). https://doi.org/10.1038/s41467-018-03399-2. This data was obtained from the OpenNeuro database. Its accession number is ds000228

17. Thielscher, A., Antunes, A., Saturnino, G.B.: Field modeling for transcranial magnetic stimulation: a useful tool to understand the physiological effects of TMS? In: 2015 37th Annual International Conference of the IEEE Engineering in Medicine and Biology Society (EMBC), August 2015, pp. 222–225. IEEE (2015)

18. Vidorreta, M., et al.: Whole-brain background-suppressed pCASL MRI with 1D-accelerated 3D RARE stack-of-spirals readout-dataset 3

Image-Processing Based Smart Refreshable Braille Display

Suresh Gobee[✉], Syed Shah Hamza Ahsan, Shankar Duraikannan,
and Vickneswari Durairajah

Asia Pacific University, TPM, 57000 Kuala Lumpur, Malaysia
{suresh.gobee,vicky_nesa}@apu.edu.my

Abstract. This project aims to make a Refreshable Braille Display which would utilize the Tesseract-OCR library with the Raspberry Pi. The available Braille displays in the market use high-end technologies to provide better accuracy, thus increasing the prices of these display mechanisms. Hence, there is a requirement for an alternative technology to display the Braille characters that are cost-efficient and easily accepted by the blind or visually impaired people. The real-time image is streamed on the webserver using the mobile application IP Webcam and then the image was pre-processed using the OpenCV functions. The overall process of the project involves Image-To-Text conversion using the Tesseract-OCR library and Converting the text recognized by the Tesseract-OCR into Braille language, also Text-To-Speech conversion is done. This Braille conversion is then displayed on the Smart Refreshable Braille Display which was deign using servo motor actuators. The Smart Refreshable Braille Display had an overall accuracy of 97%, which was evaluated through tests. This project is practical and of great use for the blind and visually impaired.

Keywords: Python-OpenCV · Raspberry Pi · Tesseract-OCR · Braille

1 Introduction

The digital revolution has not reached the same way for every human. Visually impaired and blind people are left behind as nowadays the next great inventions are to be expected to appear on the mobile phone screens. The blind people play an integral part in our societies, like everyone else, they also help in the role of its development effectively. As of 2010, the World Health Organization (WHO) estimated that there are 40 to 45 million blind people and 135 million that are visually impaired, and this number is growing every year [1].

1.1 Justification for the Research

The available Braille displays in the market use high-end technologies to provide better accuracy, thus increasing the prices of these display mechanisms. Hence, there is a

© Springer Nature Switzerland AG 2021
F. Ibrahim et al. (Eds.): ICIBEL 2019, IFMBE Proceedings 81, pp. 76–85, 2021.
https://doi.org/10.1007/978-3-030-65092-6_9

requirement for an alternative technology to display the Braille characters that are cost-efficient and easily accepted by the blind or visually impaired people. The commercially available Braille displays commonly use piezoelectric technology, these Braille display mechanisms typically (65–100 per Braille character cell) have the price range from 2500 USD–4000 USD. Hence, there is a requirement for an alternative technology to display the Braille characters that are cost-efficient and easily accepted by the blind or visually impaired people [2].

The purpose of this research is to find and create an alternative to the already existing Refreshable Braille Displays (RBD) that are expensive and can compete with them in terms of accuracy. So that it can be easily available to people who need such technologies and can play a role in building the society. Portability of the Refreshable Braille Display (RBD) is one of the most integral features, if the mechanism/ system is too heavy or complex, it will hinder the blind or visually impaired people to use this Refreshable Braille Display and would require someone to help them set it up first. Some of the most commonly used material to build the mechanism for these Braille displays use piezoelectric and solenoids/ relays. But there aren't many that combine these two aspects of using image processing and then generating output in refreshable Braille displays. This project combines both image with text recognition and converting it to braille display. [3–5] and [6].

2   Proposed Methodology

The main component in the proposed system is the Raspberry Pi which utilizes the python programming language. Figure 1 depicts the block diagram for the proposed system.

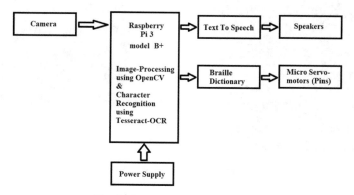

Fig. 1. Overall RDB system design

2.1   Design and Development

The Refreshable Braille Display (RBD) mechanism concept design for the prototype is developed using SolidWorks. The design has 6 dots that will be used for displaying the

Braille Characters. The concept design of the mechanism is aligned in 2 columns and 3 rows which is a requirement for displaying Braille characters as shown in Fig. 2. The dot structures and the micro servo are connected to shaft with pin joints. So, when the micro servo motors it pulls the shaft downwards which makes the pins to push up as shown in Fig. 2. The mechanism will be covered and only the pins will be pushed out as shown in Fig. 3.

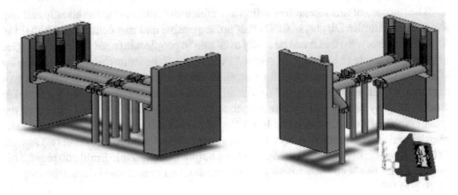

Fig. 2. Isometric view of the interior of the mechanism with the servo attached per rod

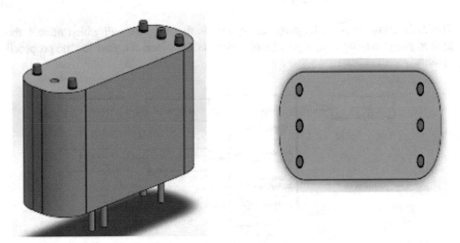

Fig. 3. Mechanism exterior

The concept design for the prototype is built using SolidWorks software and the micro servo-motors as stated above the micro servo-motors has the torque of 1.80 kg-cm and utilizes rotatory movement, which required the design to be tweaked to support the micro servo-motors rotary movements. Another reason is as the micro servo-motors can only be used for 9 g of weight. This meant the mechanism for the Braille display needed to be 3D printed and would be required to weigh less. So, the removal of some parts was necessary to achieve this threshold and reducing the density of the parts being printed.

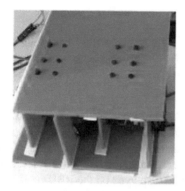 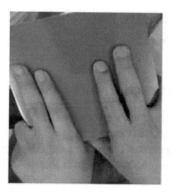

Fig. 4. Actual mechanism to display 2 characters

With the changed 3D design, it fits perfectly with the micro servo-motors and utilizes the rotary movements of the micro servo-motors to push the pins up or pull it down hence achieving the results set for the mechanism. Figure 4 shows the system can be used to display 2 braille characters at a time which are displaying the numbers and the symbols.

2.2 Constructional Diagram

The Fig. 5 illustrates the wiring diagram for the entire project. The Raspberry Pi is the brain of the system, micro servo-motors are connected to the GPIO pins of the Raspberry Pi, which controls each micro servo-motor using Pulse Width Modulation (PWM) as depicted in the micro servo-motors have 3 inputs which are for power supply, ground and pulse. The pulse input is through which the Raspberry Pi controls the micro servo-motors moving the micro servo-motors clockwise or counterclockwise as programmed in the python coding. The power supplied to each micro servo-motors is supplied from the Raspberry Pi's 5V output pin and similar for grounding the micro servo-motors to complete the circuit.

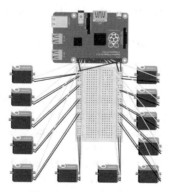

Fig. 5. Circuit diagram

2.3 Other Hardware Requirements

Apart from Raspberry Pi, a mobile camera is required for capturing the image and a speaker to transmit the audio so that the users can hear it.

3 System Software Design

The software design consists of various methods that help in achieving the results. From the conversion of the image into the text to displaying it on the Braille display. The camera captures the image which than pre-processed by utilizing the OpenCV functions and then processed by the Tesseract-OCR for the character recognition. These recognized characters are converted into Braille language ad displayed on the RBD.

3.1 Image-To-Text Conversion

The real-time image is captured using the mobile camera which sends it to the Raspberry Pi through online web server through the mobile application IP Webcam that transmits real-time images as captured from the mobile's camera. Using OpenCV library the image is pre-processed such as grey-scaling the image, OTSU Thresholding, and noise removal using the median blur filter which are the functions in OpenCV library. This pre-processed image aids in character recognition as its sets the Regions of Interests (ROI) for the Tesseract-OCR to work on which is an open-source and pre-trained library for identifying the characters from the image and can be further trained as per the requirements. Using the pytesseract (Tesseract-OCR library for Raspberry Pi) the characters are recognized from the image and converted to a string.

3.2 Text-To-Speech Synthesis

Google's Text-To-Speech (gTTS) library is being used in the system for converting the recognized characters into audio impulses. The library is pre-trained for synthesising the recognized characters, which would be grouped and spoken. It also provides with a different accent, speed of delivery and language. The library creates an audio (.wav) format file for the speakers to transmit. The VLC library is utilized for playing the audio file saved by the gTTS library over a speaker. The Raspberry Pi controller is capable of delivering audio output. The required audio output can be received via earphones or speakers through the audio jack or the HDMI port respectively.

3.3 Text-To-Braille Conversion

The characters recognized by the pytesseract is also converted into the Braille characters. This checking for input data is done using the if function in the python programming language that checks if the word recognized is an uppercase, lowercase, numerical value or a symbol and adds the identifications as per the requirements and the guidelines of writing the Braille language. This converts it into Braille characters, then it actuates the micro servo-motors as per the requirement that pushes or pulls the 3D printed Braille pins accordingly to represent a Braille character.

The Fig. 6 depicts the entire flow of the project which contains a graphical representation of how the system works from start to finish.

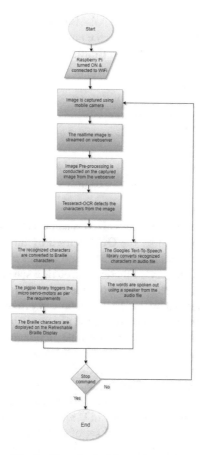

Fig. 6. Flowchart of the entire project

4 Hardware and Software Results

The results were of two types the simulation/software-based and hardware-based. The simulation/software-based covers the image processing of the input data, which was the real-time streamed images and converting to the recognized characters into Braille language. And the conversion of recognized words into the audio file. The Hardware-based result was displaying the converted Braille characters on the Smart Refreshable Braille Display (RBD) using the micro servo-motors and transmitting the audio file generated by the gTTS library. The accuracy of the Tesseract-OCR is greatly affected by the quality of the image captured, if the image captured is blurred or the pixels are not clear, even after pre-processing the image the results will not be accurate. The mobile camera captures the image of the paper and streams it on the LAN, which contain different types of characters at different sizes and fonts. This covers most of the key areas which are required for checking the accuracy of the OCR. The input data has uppercase and lowercase letters, numerical values and symbols.

The image is grey-scaled, binarized, the noise is reduced. This helps to set the Regions of Interests (ROI) for the OCR and removes the unwanted elements from the image. The characters recognized by the OCR and the Braille conversion of the characters.

Asia Pacific University of Technology & Innovation (APU)
Technology Park Malaysia
Bukit Jalil, Kuala Lumpur 57000
Malaysia

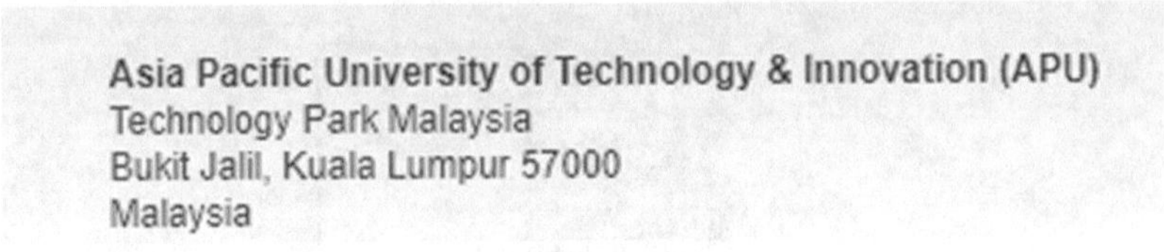

Fig. 7. Test image

As seen in Fig. 7 the characters recognized is same as the input data provided. The characters which are recognized by the OCR is used by the gTTS library's functions which converts these characters into sentences and creates an audio file which is then transmitted using the VLC library's functions through a speaker. Allowing the user to hear the characters the OCR recognized from the captured image. The Braille conversion of the characters is defined by the Braille dictionary provided in the python coding, which determined using the if function in python programming language which checks the characters which are recognized with the Braille dictionary and then prints the counterpart of the character with the indicators where there is a requirement to differentiate the uppercase and lowercase alphabets, numerical values and symbols. The Smart RBD working, displaying the characters. The character being displayed is "a" which is represented by "·" in Braille language which is the first pin in the cell. The first pin is raised above all the others displaying the letter "a" in Braille. Each character recognized by the OCR is displayed on it, with an additional set of cells that helps in differentiating the uppercase and lowercase alphabets, numerical values and symbols.

5   Discussion- Project Findings and Testing

The tests were conducted for evaluating the project's accuracy and aspects which can affect the performance of the OCR and the Braille display. The project was tested based on the following:

5.1   Testing for the Accuracy of the OCR Depending on the Distance and Length of Characters

The test was conducted to find the accuracy of the Tesseract-OCR based on the font size of the characters. To evaluate the distance at which the OCR could not recognize the characters. The results provided with the distance at which the mobile camera should be placed or the ideal location for getting the most accurate results. Table 1 shows the testing results.

Table 1. OCR accuracy depending on the distance

Distance (cm)	No. of characters recognized	Font size of the character not recognized (cm)	Accuracy (%)
10	149	–	100
12	149	–	100
15	148	0.3 or 10pt	99.33
20	145	0.3 or 10pt	97.32
25	144	0.3 or 10pt	96.64
30	139	0.3 or 10pt	93.29
40	139	0.3 or 10pt	93.29

5.2 Testing for the Accuracy of the Braille Display

The test was conducted to find the accuracy of the RBD. To verify that the characters recognized by the OCR which are then converted into Braille language will be displayed correctly on the Smart Refreshable Braille Display (RBD). The results provided the accuracy of the RBD which was felt by the participants of the test. Table 2 shows the testing results. Participants were based on the availability and willingness to be experimented upon.

Table 2. Accuracy of the RBD

Participant	No. of character recognized	Accuracy (%)
Sample 1	34	100
Sample 2	33	97.06
Sample 3	33	97.06
Sample 4	34	100
Sample 5	34	100
Sample 6	33	97.06
Sample 7	34	100
Sample 8	34	100

5.3 Testing for the Refresh Rate of the OCR

The test was conducted to check the time it takes for the OCR to detect the characters from the input data and whether the number of characters affects the time it takes by the OCR to recognize the characters from the image. The results provided with the time taken by the OCR to recognize the characters. Table 3 shows the testing results.

Table 3. Time taken by the OCR to recognize the characters

No. of characters in the image	Time taken to recognize the characters (Seconds)
12	5
31	8
111	18
146	20
1283	166

In every project, there will be some discrepancy between theoretical and experimental results. These might occur due to many factors; hence it is important to design a system which can be adjusted to achieve the theoretical or the experimental results are considered to be accomplishing the objectives.

In this section, the theoretical and experimental results will be compared to see if the desired result from the ideal case for the recognized characters which is of 100% accuracy is achieved by the OCR. As shown in Sect. 5.1, the system has an overall 97% accuracy which is not an ideal percentage of 100%, but the factors that affect the accuracy of the OCR can be identified as lighting and distance from the sample. The environmental lighting also plays a major role in image processing if the room is too dark, the image captured by the mobile camera is blurred and noisy, therefore when filtered using the OpenCV library it is not considered characters, this can be eliminated by providing at least Lux of 1000 which is normal room lighting when using the project.

6   Conclusion and Recommendation

The mechanism can use different servo-motors that are smaller than micro servo-motors used for the project such as sub-micro servo-motors 3.7 g which will reduce the space between the Braille pins thus only one finger would be required for detecting the Braille characters instead of the two fingers which are required for this Smart Refreshable Braille Display (RBD). The limitation of using the IP Webcam mobile application is that the mobile application is only available on Android platform, therefore if the users have some other mobile Operating System (OS) the application will not be available for them. So, using an application that covers all the OS. The language used for the character recognition for this project was English which can be changed to support other languages such as French, Urdu and Malay.

References

1. World Health Organisation: World Health Organisation (2018). https://www.who.int/news-room/fact-sheets/detail/blindness-and-visual-impairment. Accessed 5th Mar 2019
2. Sapra, P., Parsurampuria, A.K., Gupta, D., Muralikrishnan, S., Raj, M., Anand, A., Darda, V., Paul, R., Balakrishnan, M., Rao, P.V.M.: A compliant mechanism design for refreshable Braille display using shape memory alloy. In: 2015 ASME/IEEE International Conference on Mechatronic and Embedded Systems and Applications, Boston, 2nd–5th August 2015, p. 10 (2015)

3. Raghunandan, A., Anuradha, M.R.: The methods used in text to Braille conversion and vice versa. Int. J. Innov. Res. Comput. Commun. Eng. (IJIRCCE) **5**(3), 5297–5310 (2017)
4. Schmidt, M.B., Metzger, L.G., Mortimer, R., Ramirez, A.R.G.: New user interface based on a single Braille cell. Informática na Educação: Teoria & Prática **20**(2), 157–168 (2017)
5. Shahriman, A.S., Wahid, M.A., Saad, S.M., Zain, M.Z.MD., Hussein, M., Ahmad, Z., Yaacob, M.S., Abdullah, M.Y., Mohamad, M.: Improving design of piezoelectric braille cell for Braille display devices. J. Telecommun. Electron. Comput. Eng. (JTEC) **10**(1–14), 107–111 (2018)
6. Sutariya, R.D., Singh, H.S., Babariya, S.R., Kadiyar, S.A., Modi, D.H.: Refreshable Braille display for the visually impaired. In: 2017 14th IEEE India Council International Conference (INDICON), Roorkee, 15th–17th December 2017, pp. 1–5 (2017)

Metamaterial Applicator for Hyperthermia Cancer Treatment Procedure: Overview Study

Vei Ling Wong$^{(\boxtimes)}$ ⓘ and Kasumawati Lias ⓘ

Faculty of Engineering, Universiti Malaysia Sarawak (UNIMAS), 94300 Kota Samarian, Sarawak, Malaysia
veilingwong@gmail.com, lkasumati@unimas.my

Abstract. This paper presents an overview of metamaterial slabs or lens as an integrated structure for applicators used in hyperthermia cancer treatment procedure. Hyperthermia treatment procedure (HTP) is a new technique that exposes a cancerous tissue by increasing tissue temperature until 41 °C to 45 °C at a certain period with electromagnetic radiation. Based on the previous study, by moving the microwave sources relative to the metamaterial (MTM) lenses from a tumor/cancer phantom alters the concentration of heating within biological tissue. In this paper, the overview of a metamaterial study on HTP from 2009 to 2019 was carried out. This study indicated that the left-handed metamaterial (LHM) lens was observed to be able to improve the focusing capabilities of HTP on the treated tissue. However, a further study is significantly required to provide different focus position distances on the treated tissue for different stages of cancer. Therefore, a modified HTP applicator integration with an MTM lens structure was proposed. It is aimed to improve focus position distance on the treated tissue and to reduce unwanted hot-spots on surrounding healthy tissues simultaneously. The proposed modified structure was presented in this paper. Specific absorption rate (SAR) simulation was carried out with SEMCAD X 14.8.4 to obtain a SAR distribution for determining penetration depth and focusing position distance on the treated tissue.

Keywords: Metamaterial lens · Hyperthermia · Left-handed metamaterial · Specific absorption rate

1 Introduction

In recent years, hyperthermia treatment procedure (HTP) applicators for non-invasive HTP have been extensively studied. HTP, an alternative therapy for cancer [1], is often used as adjuvant therapy with chemotherapy and radiotherapy [2]. HTP is a technique to expose cancerous tissue with electromagnetic (EM) radiation in order to increase tissue temperatures within 41 °C–45 °C at a certain period. Based on the previous research, it was observed that this hyperthermia technique converts cancerous tissues into necrotic tissues and destroys cancerous tissues with minimal side effects [1, 3, 4].

Generally, HTP can be either invasive or noninvasive, depending on the location of HTP applicators, which are either inserted into or on the surface of the human body.

© Springer Nature Switzerland AG 2021
F. Ibrahim et al. (Eds.): ICIBEL 2019, IFMBE Proceedings 81, pp. 86–92, 2021.
https://doi.org/10.1007/978-3-030-65092-6_10

Invasive HTP can be much more effective than a non-invasive HTP, as it is pointed and inserted directly to the targeted region [5]. However, invasive HTP can cause several adverse health effects, such as bleeding during minor surgery, which is required in treatment application.

Non-invasive HTP, adverse health effects can be minimized as it does not require minor surgery. Non-invasive HTP is simpler to handle than invasive HTP and is suitable for use as an in-situ applicator [1, 4]. However, poor penetration depth and focus position distance are the main drawbacks of noninvasive HTP.

In conjunction, MTM structure is integrated into the base antenna to form a modified HTP applicator. The main objective of this integration is to improve penetration depth and focus position distance on the treated tissue resulted from the existing HTP applicator.

2 Metamaterial Applicator in HTP

Current research proved that concentration of heating is adjustable by moving microwave sources with respect to MTM lenses based on tumor position [6, 7]. MTM classification was first proposed by Veselago in 1968 as an artificial component, which consists of negative permittivity, ε and permeability, μ. This type of MTM is known as the left-handed material (LHM) and acts as a negative refractive index (NRI) lens to induce electromagnetic field (EMF) from an energy source [8].

The two commonly used MTM structures are electrical dipoles or a thin wires array and the magnetic loops or split-ring resonators array (SRR) [9].

The thin wires array (Fig. 1 [a]) is also known as epsilon-negative (ENG) MTM. Through the parallel configuration of thin metallic wire meshes, ENG MTM will exhibits high-pass properties for the incoming plane waves. The wires are parallel to the electric field and perform a negative effect of permittivity below the plasma frequency. The wire can be made of silver, gold, aluminum, or copper [9].

Split-ring resonators (Fig. 1 [b]), the most used structure in designing mu-negative (MNG) MTM. An SRR cell, which consisted of two concentric metallic rings (either square or circle) forming an array structure by a specific gap, d. The gap between the inner and outer rings shows capacitive effects, while each ring itself becomes inductive. Thus, the integration of the two rings forms an LC resonance circuit [9].

ENG and MNG MTMs can be combined to form a double-negative (DNG) material (Fig. 1 [c]), which is known as negative refractive index (NRI) material. NRI materials contribute to the negative permittivity effect from wire arrays and negative permeability of SRR array [9].

DNG MTMs are frequency-dependent, which results in the refractive index n. This is explainable by Drude-Lorentz models, which are indicated in Eqs. 1, 2, and 3 [9].

$$n \equiv n_{eff}(\omega) = \sqrt{\varepsilon_{eff}(\omega)\mu_{eff}(\omega)} \tag{1}$$

$$\varepsilon_{eff}(\omega) = 1 - \frac{\omega_{ep}^2 - \omega_{e0}^2}{\omega^2 - \omega_{e0}^2 - j\omega\gamma_c} \tag{2}$$

$$\mu_{eff}(\omega) = 1 - \frac{F\omega^2}{\omega^2 - \omega_{m0}^2 - j\omega\Gamma} \tag{3}$$

where $\varepsilon_{eff}(\omega)$, $\mu_{eff}(\omega)$, ω_{ep}, ω_{mp}, ω_{e0}, ω_{m0}, γ_c, F, and Γ are frequency-dependent effective permittivity, frequency dependent effective permeability, electric plasma frequency, magnetic plasma frequencies, electric resonant frequency, magnetic resonant frequency, collision frequency, amplitude factor and damping factor, respectively.

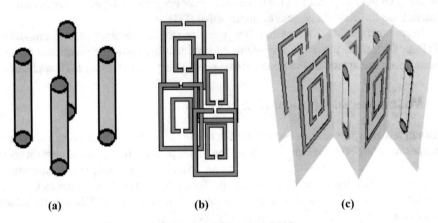

(a)   (b)   (c)

Fig. 1. (a) ENG, (b) MNG and (c) DNG structure

2.1   Current MTM Slabs or Lens Research in HTP

Since Pendry's publication titled *negative refraction makes a perfect lens* in the year 2000 [10], the investigation of NRI material was inspired. From [10], this perfect lens, or as mentioned by Pendry as "superlens", can be achieved with the microwave band of current technology [10, 11]. In [11], Pendry's works were further elaborated, and the concept of MTM was implemented along with the introduces of the Pendry-Veselago slab lens. These investigations made it possible to obtain unique effects, such as imaging with subwavelength image resolution, which is generated through NRI that supports a host of surface plasmon states for both polarizations of light.

Thus, starting from this remarkable study, investigations on MTMs in antenna development have increased, as well as HTP for cancer treatment. This is because of perfect lens or more known as left-handed material (LHM) provides substantial EM energy-focusing capability on the treated tissue [12]. Table 1 presents an overview of MTM slabs or lens research from 2009 to 2019.

Table 1. Overview of MTM slabs or lens researches

Published year and reference	Type of structure	Targeted organ	Research finding(s)
2009, [13]	DNG – LHM slabs	Muscle	When the source was moving towards the LHM lens, the heating depth was increased. Higher input power was required to archive the necessary therapeutic temperature
2009, [14]	Combination of dielectric filling and metamaterial layer	Brain	The combined structure increased system response to the relative movements of the head around a geometrical focal point
2010, [15]	DNG - Γ-Shaped LHM Lens	Breast	Incoming sources were applied to horizontal, vertical, or both sides of Γ-shaped LHM lens. The condition with only single-sided sources reduced hyperthermia performance
2011, [16]	DNG- metallic slabs with broadside-coupled split-ring resonators	Breast	SAR was focused on the targeted tissue region
2014, [17]	DNG - metamaterial zeroth order (ZOR) mode resonator (lumped LC circuit)	Muscle	The proposed structure generated good EM waves penetration depth towards biological tissue
2015, [7]	DNG – single, double and conformal four lens LHM structure	Breast	The conformal four-lens showed better focusing resolution and temperature concentration within the tumor than single and double lens. Due to poor longitudinal resolution, single-lens LHM could not achieve good hyperthermia performance
2016, [18]	DNG - metamaterial ZOR mode resonator (lumped LC circuit)	Muscle	Composition of ZOR array structures radiated EM waves that were nearly plane waves in structure. The shape of the heating pattern was adjustable by manipulating relative power to ZOR structures
2019, [12]	DNG – cylindrical and flat LHM lens	Breast	Cylindrical LHM lens showed better focusing effect than flat rectangular LHM lens

3   Proposed Design

The proposed design for this research is provided in Fig. 2.

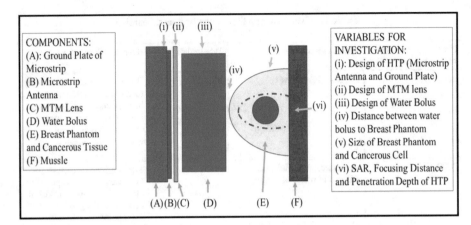

Fig. 2. Proposed modified HTP

As illustrated in Fig. 2, HTP applicator is a combination of two main components: microstrip antenna and MTM lens. Water bolus is then added to the treatment procedure to complement the HTP execution. The HTP applicator contributes an important role in the treatment as it is used to radiate thermal energy or heat to the targeted tissue. This HTP applicator is noninvasive, which applies externally to the human body.

Since this research experimentation is mainly conducted through simulation, the research tool, which is selected to be used is known as SEMCAD X 14.8.4 produced by SPEAG. SEMCAD X is a highly specialized full-wave EMF solver used to design HTP applicators and determine radiation distribution, which presents the EM energy penetration depth and its energy focus distance.

Various MTM structures are investigated in order to observe the effects on the focus position distance on the treated tissue. SAR simulation is conducted to determine the penetration depth and focus position depth.

According to the standard of International Electrotechnical Commission (IEC) and Institute of Electrical and Electronics Engineers (IEEE), IEC/IEEE 62704-1, SAR can be calculated by Formulas 4, 5, and 6,

$$SAR = \frac{\delta}{\delta t}\left(\frac{\delta W}{\rho \delta V}\right) \tag{4}$$

When implemented to the electric field,

$$SAR = \frac{\sigma E^2}{2\rho} \tag{5}$$

Therefore, based on electric field distribution, SAR can be related to the increase in temperature at a given point as in the formula below.

$$SAR = \frac{c\Delta T}{\Delta t}\bigg|t = 0, \tag{6}$$

where, $W, t, V, E, \rho, T, \sigma$, and c stand for energy absorbed (W), time taken (sec), volume of element (m^3), peak electric field vector (V/m), density of element (kg/m^3), temperature (°C), conductivity of tissue (S/m), and specific heat capacity (J/kg°C) respectively.

These modifications and integration processes are aimed at improving focus position distance at different stages of cancer.

4 Conclusion

HTP is an alternative treatment for cancer treatment procedure by using induced heat and form the biological effect. The effectiveness of HTP is significantly depended on focusing position distance of the energy in order to elevate the temperature of the cancerous tissue within 41 °C–45 °C. HTP denatures cancerous tissues into necrotic tissues and destroys them with minimal side effects. In this overview study, MTM or LHM lens had shown a good capability to provide penetration depth and EM energy focus position distance on treated tissues. However, in terms of focus position distance, this technique needs improvement to cater to different stages of cancer. Thus, this research was carried out to introduce a modified HTP applicator that can improve focus position distance at different stages of cancer.

Acknowledgment. The authors would like to thank the Faculty of Engineering, Universiti Malaysia Sarawak for the support.

References

1. Lias, K.B., Zulkarnaen, M., Narihan, A., Buniyamin, N.: An antenna with an embedded EBG structure for non invasive hyperthermia cancer treatment. In: 2014 IEEE Conference on Biomedical Engineering and Sciences (2014). https://doi.org/10.1109/IECBES.2014.704 7577
2. Koo, Y.S., Kazemi, R., Liu, Q., Phillips, J.C., Fathy, A.E.: Development of a high SAR conformal antenna for hyperthermia tumors treatment. IEEE Trans. Antennas Propag. **62**, 5830–5840 (2014). https://doi.org/10.1109/TAP.2014.2357419
3. Korkmaz, E., Isik, O., Kara, S.: Electromagnetic modeling of a female breast hyperthermia applicator. In: IEEE Antennas and Propagation Society, AP-S International Symposium (Digest), pp. 2048–2049 (2013). https://doi.org/10.1109/APS.2013.6711682
4. Sharma, N., Jain, B., Singla, P., Prasad, R.R.: Rectangular patch microstrip antenna: a survey. Int. Adv. Res. J. Sci. Eng. Technol. **1**, 144–147 (2014). https://iarjset.com/wp-content/uploads/2014/12/IARJSET15-a-pradeepsingla-RECTANGULAR-PATCH-MICRO-STRIP-ANTENNA-A-SURVEY.pdf
5. Wang, L., Yin, D., Li, M., Li, L.: Microstrip near-field focusing for microwave non-invasive breast cancer thermotherapy. In: 2014 31th URSI General Assembly and Scientific Symposium, URSI GASS 2014, pp. 1–4 (2014). https://doi.org/10.1109/URSIGASS.2014.693 0098
6. Jaffar, N.A., Lias, K.B., Madzhi, N.K., Buniyamin, N.: An overview of metamaterials used in applicators in hyperthermia cancer treatment procedure. In: 2017 International Conference on Electrical, Electronics and System Engineering, ICEESE 2017 2018-Janua, pp. 32–36 (2018). https://doi.org/10.1109/ICEESE.2017.8298389

7. Leggio, L., De Varona, O., Dadrasnia, E.: A comparison between different schemes of microwave cancer hyperthermia treatment by means of left-handed metamaterial lenses. Prog. Electromagn. Res. **150**, 73–87 (2015). https://doi.org/10.2528/PIER14101408

8. Freire, M.J., Marques, R.: Metamaterial focusing device for microwave hyperthermia. Microw. Opt. Technol. Lett. **53**, 2868–2872 (2011). https://doi.org/10.1002/mop.26434

9. Wojciech, J.K., Thanh, N.C.: Metamaterials in application to improve antenna parameters, metamaterials and metasurfaces (chap 4). In: Josep, C.F. (ed.) IntechOpen (2019). https://doi.org/10.5772/intechopen.80636

10. Pendry, J.B.: Negative refraction makes a perfect lens. Phys. Rev. Lett. **85**, 3966–3969 (2000). https://doi.org/10.1103/PhysRevLett.85.3966

11. Guenneau, S., Ramakrishna, S.A.: Negative refractive index, perfect lenses and checkerboards: trapping and imaging effects in folded optical spaces. Comptes Rendus Phys. **10**, 352–378 (2009). https://doi.org/10.1016/j.crhy.2009.04.002

12. Jaffar, N.A., Lias, K., Madzhi, N.K., Buniyamin, N., Member, I.: Improving the performance of applicators for use in hyperthermia cancer treatment procedure by the introduction of LHM lens. Int. J. Electr. Electron. Syst. Res. **14**, 697–705 (2019). https://jeesr.uitm.edu.my/v1/IEESR/Vol.14/article5.pdf

13. Gong, Y., Wang, G.: Superficial tumor hyperthermia with flat left-handed metamaterial lens. Prog. Electromagn. Res. **98**, 389–405 (2009). https://doi.org/10.2528/PIER09091401

14. Karathanasis, K.T., Gouzouasis, I.A., Karanasiou, I.S., Uzunoglu, N.K.: The use of left handed materials for the optimization of the focusing attributes of a biomedical hybrid system. In: 2009 International Symposium on Electromagnetic Compatibility - EMC Europe, pp. 1–4 (2009). https://doi.org/10.1109/EMCEUROPE.2009.5189679

15. Tao, Y., Wang, G.: Influence of source offset on breast tumor hyperthermia with Γ-shaped LHM lens applicator. 2010 International Conference on Microwave and Millimeter Wave Technology, ICMMT 2010, pp. 1859–1861 (2010). https://doi.org/10.1109/ICMMT.2010.5524876

16. Velazquez-Ahumada, M.C., Freire, M.J., Marques, R.: Metamaterial applicator for microwave hyperthermia. In: 2011 30th URSI General Assembly and Scientific Symposium (2011). https://doi.org/10.1109/URSIGASS.2011.6050641

17. Vrba, D., Vrba, J., Stauffer, P.: Novel microwave applicators based on zero-order mode resonance for hyperthermia treatment of cancer novel microwave applicators based on zero-order mode resonance for hyperthermia treatment of cancer. In: 2014 IEEE Benjamin Franklin Symposium on Microwave and Antenna Sub-Systems for Radar, Telecommunications, and Biomedical Applications (BenMAS) (2014). https://doi.org/10.1109/BenMAS.2014.7529479

18. Vrba, D., Rodrigues, D.B., Vrba, J., Stauffer, P.R.: Metamaterial antenna arrays for improved uniformity of microwave hyperthermia treatments. Prog. Electromagn. Res. **156**, 1–12 (2016). https://doi.org/10.2528/PIER16012702

Theme: Biomechanics, Ergonomics and Rehabilitation

Evaluation of CR2-Haptic Movement Quality Assessment Module for Hand

Kang Xiang Khor[1,2]([✉]), Patrick Jun Hua Chin[1], Che Fai Yeong[1,2],
Eileen Lee Ming Su[1], Aqilah Leela T. Narayanan[3], Hisyam Abdul Rahman[4],
Najib bin Abdullah[1], Muhammad Farhan bin Mustar[1], Yvonne Yee Woon Khor[3,5,6],
Hadafi Fitri Mohd Latip[3,5,6], Qamer Iqbal Khan[7], Yashitha Devi Silvadorai[7],
Tracy Chan[7], and Nimalan Arumugam[7]

[1] School of Electrical Engineering, Faculty of Engineering, Universiti Teknologi Malaysia (UTM), 81300 Skudai, Johor, Malaysia
xiangkk@gmail.com, cfyeong@utm.my
[2] Center of Artificial Intelligence and Robotics, UTM, 54100 Kuala Lumpur, Malaysia
[3] School of Biomedical Engineering and Health Science, Faculty of Engineering, UTM, 81300 Skudai, Johor, Malaysia
[4] Universiti Tun Hussein Onn Malaysia, 86400 Parit Raja, Johor, Malaysia
[5] Sports Innovation and Technology Centre, UTM, 81300 Skudai, Johor, Malaysia
[6] Institute of Human Centered Engineering (iHumEn), UTM, 81310 Skudai, Johor, Malaysia
[7] National Stroke Association of Malaysia (NASAM), 46050 Petaling Jaya, Selangor, Malaysia

Abstract. Objective assessment is crucial in the rehabilitation process for physiotherapists to determine the progress of the patient and to provide the best treatment in therapy. However, current rehabilitations rely heavily on manual labour and lack objective assessments, as well as quantitative diagnosis and evaluation. This project aims to evaluate the movement assessment modules of CR2-Haptic, a portable and reconfigurable rehabilitation robot that can be used to provide an objective assessment for the targeted movement of upper limb. Both wrist and forearm movement performance were assessed in the study. Centre-out-point-to-point (CO-PTP) approach was used in the movement quality assessment module of CR2-Haptic and the proposed coordination score showed high correlation with four kinematic variables of the movement including total trial time which has the strongest relation with r^2 value of 0.85, followed by smoothness ($r^2 = 0.80$), mean velocity ($r^2 = 0.78$) and path ratio ($r^2 = 0.70$).

Keywords: Rehabilitation robotic · Assessment · Stroke · Upper limb

1 Introduction

In Malaysia, stroke is the second leading cause of death and third leading cause of severe disability [1] and every year 15 million stroke cases occur worldwide [2]. Objective assessment is crucial in the stroke rehabilitation process to determine actual progress of patient, to identify optimal rehabilitation level that patient need to embark on, and to provide the best outcome in therapy [3]. However, current rehabilitations rely heavily

© Springer Nature Switzerland AG 2021
F. Ibrahim et al. (Eds.): ICIBEL 2019, IFMBE Proceedings 81, pp. 95–102, 2021.
https://doi.org/10.1007/978-3-030-65092-6_11

on manual labour and lack objective assessments, as well as quantitative diagnosis and evaluation [4]. Robotic devices can be a good alternative, as it can accurately assess the patient's performance by using sensors [5–8]. However, most of the robots assess a combination of joints, which do not allow the identification of targeted joint performance [9]. There is a need to develop an assessment program that provides targeted joint movement to better analyse the performance of the patient in specific muscle joint. Wrist component is important to be rehabilitated, as the impairment of wrist can cause substantial dysfunctions of the hand motion and consequently, of the entire upper extremity [10]. Many functional gains are more dependent on wrist and hand movements than on the mobility of shoulder and elbow [11]. Thus, this project aims to evaluate the movement quality assessment modules of CR2-Haptic targeted for wrist movement [12].

2   Methods

Centre-out-point-to-point (CO-PTP) approach was used in the movement quality assessment module of CR2-Haptic, as it can be used to determine the most aspect of movement quality compared to other approach including the temporal efficiency, ease of movement, smoothness, efficacy, and movement efficiency [9]. Temporal efficiency is defined to be the optimal time taken to complete the task and the time taken is expected to be reduced with patient's recovery [9]. Therefore, reaching time and stabilization time are used to evaluate the temporal efficiency of the subject movement. Reaching time (RT) is the time taken between initial target position to reach within the tolerance of target. Total trial time (TT) is the total time taken to complete the movement within the set tolerance. Stabilization time (ST) is the differences between the reaching time and the time when the hand remained in the tolerance area for 1 s.

The measure of efficiency in movement is indicated by the use of the shortest trajectory from the initial position to reach the target. The extra length in trajectories indicate the use of other movement strategies and indicate the greater energy expenditure than normal movement pattern [13]. Path length (PL) and path ratio (PR) are used to determine the movement efficiency. The path length was measured based on the Eq. 4. Actual path length (APL) is the total accumulated distance along the movement from initial position until the user reaches the target. Ideal path length (IPL) is the shortest distance between the initial position and the final target. Path ratio is the ratio between the total distance travelled from movement onset to movement offset and task ideal distance as shown in Eq. 5.

Mean velocity (MV) was used to determine the ease of movement, which is defined as the ability to complete the movement with the least efforts. Higher mean velocity reflects the decrease of abnormal effort to perform the required movement. The mean velocity is calculated by using the actual path length divided by total trial time as shown in the Eq. 6. Post-stroke patients normally will have jagged movements composed of a series of short and rapid sub-movements, representing a complete or near-complete stop between each apparent sub-movement. These jagged movements will be reflected as change in velocity over time and can be evaluated by measuring the number of zero crossing in acceleration profile.

Figure 1 shows the experimental setup and movement assessment program interface. During the assessment, the subjects will be directed to hit the pre-set target as fast as possible with minimal jerk. The targets set are ranged from $-30°$ to $30°$. The target sequence will start from neutral position, $0° > 20° > 0° > -20° > 0° > 30° > -30° > 0$. The movement position of the user will be recorded and processed. The data were collected from two post-stroke subjects (S2 and S7) in study [14] and three healthy subjects. The two stroke subjects were assessed before and after the treatment.

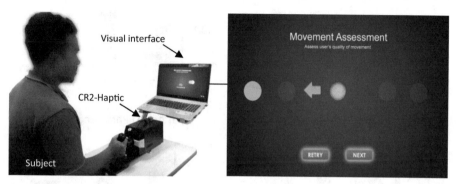

Fig. 1. Experimental setup. CR2-Haptic movement assessment with subject (left) and movement assessment software interface (right).

Kinematic variables were extracted from the recorded data during the movement coordination assessment. Objective assessment on movement quality and the variables were used to validate the developed coordination score formula. The movement quality assessment is determined by using the coordination score as shown in Eq. 1, which is comprised of timer (see Eq. 2) and movement score (see Eq. 3).

$$Coordination\ score,\ CS = 0.5\ (timer\ score) + 0.5\ (movement\ score) \tag{1}$$

$$Timer\ score = -0.125\ (total\ time\ used) + 1.25 \tag{2}$$

$$Movement\ Score = \left(\frac{Target - Initial\ Position}{Total\ distance\ travelled}\right)^2 \tag{3}$$

$$Path\ Length\ (PL) = \sum_{i=1}^{N-1} \sqrt{(\theta_{i+1} - \theta_i)^2} \tag{4}$$

$$Path\ Ratio\ (PR) = \frac{actual\ path\ length\ (APL)}{ideal\ path\ length\ (IPL)} \times 100\% \tag{5}$$

$$Mean\ Velocity\ (MV) = \frac{actual\ path\ length\ (APL)}{total\ time\ used} \tag{6}$$

Four kinematic variables including total trial time, smoothness, mean velocity and path ratio) were used to compare with coordination score to determine the correlation between the variables and the developed coordination score. Ethical approval for the study was obtained from the National Stroke Association of Malaysia (NASAM) Institutional Review Board; the clinical trial registration number was NCT02274675.

3 Results

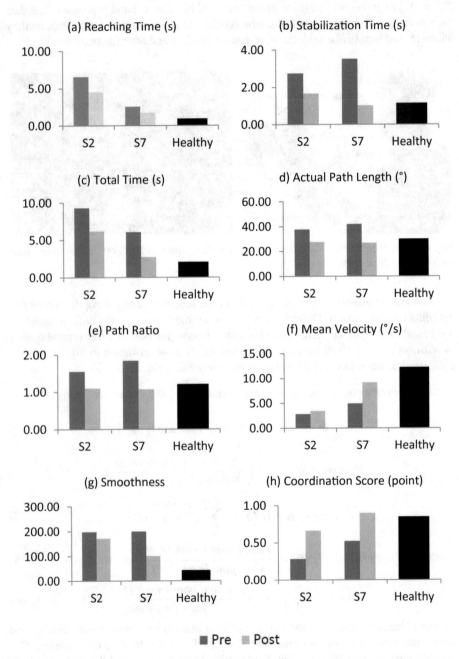

Fig. 2. Correlation of kinematic variables with coordination score in assessment module of CR2-Haptic. (a) Total trial time, (b) smoothness, (c) mean velocity and (d) path ratio.

Figure 2 shows the results of different kinematic variables used to assess the quality of movement for S2 and S7 compared to healthy subjects' data for pronation movement. The kinematic variables include reaching time (RT), stabilization time (ST) total trial time (TT), total distance travelled (TD), path ratio (PR), mean velocity (MV), smoothness

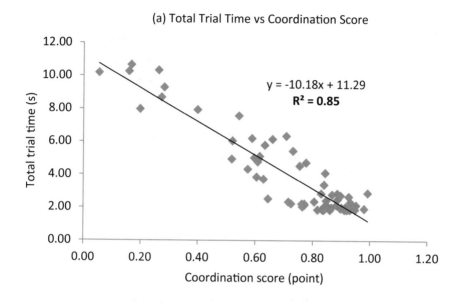

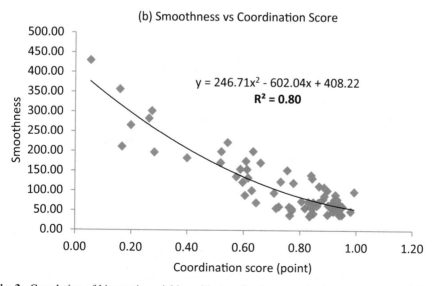

Fig. 3. Correlation of kinematic variables with coordination score in the assessment module of CR2-Haptic. (a) Total trial time and (b) smoothness.

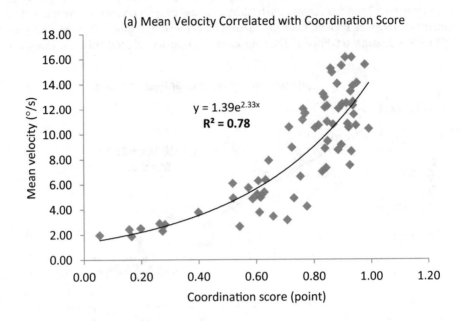

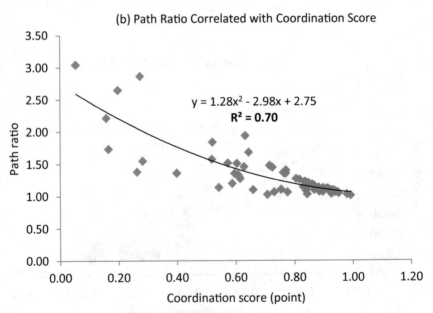

Fig. 4. Correlation of kinematic variables with coordination score in the assessment module of CR2-Haptic. (a) mean velocity and (d) path ratio.

(SN), and coordination score (CS) for S2, S7 and the average value for three healthy subjects as a benchmark. The result shows the average value for targets at 20° and 30°.

Both subjects S2 and S7 improved in every kinematic variable. S7 performance was better than S2 in all kinematic variables. S7's stabilization time, actual path length, path ratio and coordination score were better than the healthy subject benchmark. Subject S7 was considered to achieve almost full recovery in that particular tested movement.

Figure 3 and Fig. 4 shows the correlation graph between total trial time, smoothness, mean velocity and path ratio with coordination score. Four kinematic variables were used to compare with the coordination score to determine the correlation between the variables and the developed coordination score. Total time was the combination of reaching and stabilization time. Path ratio was correlated with the actual path length. The adjusted r^2 value for all value is greater than 0.7, denoting strong correlations. Results show that total trial time has the strongest relation with r^2 value of 0.85, followed by smoothness ($r^2 = 0.80$), mean velocity ($r^2 = 0.78$) and path ratio ($r^2 = 0.70$).

4 Discussion

The results of kinematic variables from the movement assessment showed the ability of CR2-Haptic to extract the detail analysis of movement quality in terms of reaching time, stabilization time, total trial time, actual path length, path ratio, mean velocity smoothness and coordination score in pronation movement. The advantage of using this reconfigurable robot is the ability to target specific individual joint training and assessment, typically available in costly exoskeleton robot [15, 16]. The center-out point-to-point (CO-PTP) [17] had been further proven in this research which can be used to reflect improvement in robot-assisted therapy [9] interventions by using kinetic sensors.

High r^2 value between the proposed coordination score with the tested kinematic variables means this score can be used as an assessment to reflect the movement quality of the subject. It shows the developed coordination score contribute to classifying the information of different kinematic parameters describing the movement quality. However, a bigger sample size is required for further evaluation of the score. The correlation of the coordination score with clinical score should also be further investigated to determine the relationship of sub-movement to existing clinical assessment.

5 Conclusion

This study shows the developed coordination score used in movement assessment module of CR2-Haptic has strong correlation with four kinematic variable that reflect the movement quality performance; total trial time ($r^2 = 0.85$), smoothness ($r^2 = 0.80$), mean velocity ($r^2 = 0.78$) and path ratio ($r^2 = 0.70$). Hence, the CR2-Haptic with its coordination score can be used to assess movement quality of a user.

Acknowledgements. The authors would like to express their gratitude to National Stroke Association of Malaysia (NASAM), Ministry of Education (MOE), Malaysia and Biofit Technologies & Services for the contribution to the work. This work is supported by the Universiti Teknologi Malaysia research grant [04H66, 06H86, 04G42, 16H47], and Collaborative Research in Engineering, Science and Teknologi Center (CREST) R&D grant [P37C2-13].

References

1. Kooi Cheah, W., Peng Hor, C., Abdul Aziz, Z., Looi, I.: A review of stroke research in Malaysia from 2000–2014. Med. J. Malaysia **71**(1), 58–69 (2016)
2. Akhavan Hejazi, S.M., Mazlan, M., Abdullah, S.J.F., Engkasan, J.P.: Cost of post-stroke outpatient care in Malaysia. Singapore Med. J. **56**(2), 116–119 (2015)
3. Metzger, J.-C., et al.: Assessment-driven selection and adaptation of exercise difficulty in robot-assisted therapy: a pilot study with a hand rehabilitation robot. J. Neuroeng. Rehabil. **11**(1), 154 (2014)
4. Gilmore, G., Jog, M.: Future perspectives: assessment tools and rehabilitation in the new age. In: Movement Disorders Rehabilitation (2016)
5. Rahman, H.A., Xiang, K.K., Fai, Y.C., Ming, E.S.L., Narayanan, A.L.T.: Robotic assessment modules for upper limb stroke assessment: preliminary study. J. Med. Imaging Heal. Inform. **6**(1), 157–162 (2016)
6. Sen, S.L., Xiang, Y.B., Ming, E.S.L., Xiang, K.K., Fai, Y.C., Khan, Q.I.: Enhancing effectiveness of virtual reality rehabilitation system: Durian Runtuh. In: 2015 10th Asian Control Conference: Emerging Control Techniques for a Sustainable World, ASCC 2015, pp. 1–6 (2015)
7. Rahman, H.A., Khor, K.X., Yeong, C.F., Su, E.L.M., Narayanan, A.L.T.: The potential of iRest in measuring the hand function performance of stroke patients. Biomed. Mater. Eng. **28**(2), 105–116 (2017)
8. Khor, K.X., et al.: Smart balance board to improve balance and reduce fall risk: pilot study. In: IFMBE Proceedings, vol. 67 (2018)
9. Nordin, N., Xie, S.Q., Wunsche, B.: Assessment of movement quality in robot- assisted upper limb rehabilitation after stroke: a review. J. Neuroeng. Rehabil. **11**(1), 137 (2014)
10. Skirven, T.M.: Rehabilitation of the Hand and Upper Extremity, 6th edn. Elsevier Mosby, Philadelphia (2011)
11. Maciejasz, P., Eschweiler, J., Gerlach-Hahn, K., Jansen-Troy, A., Leonhardt, S.: A survey on robotic devices for upper limb rehabilitation. J. Neuroeng. Rehabil. **11**(1), 3 (2014)
12. Khor, K.X., Chin, P.J.H., Hisyam, A.R., Yeong, C.F., Narayanan, A.L.T., Su, E.L.M.: Development of CR2-Haptic: a compact and portable rehabilitation robot for wrist and forearm training. In: IECBES 2014, Conference Proceedings - 2014 IEEE Conference on Biomedical Engineering and Sciences: "Miri, Where Engineering in Medicine and Biology and Humanity Meet", pp. 424–429 (2015)
13. Colombo, R., et al.: Assessing mechanisms of recovery during robot-aided neurorehabilitation of the upper limb. Neurorehabil. Neural Repair **22**(1), 50–63 (2008)
14. Khor, K.X., et al.: Portable and reconfigurable wrist robot improves hand function for post-stroke subjects. IEEE Trans. Neural Syst. Rehabil. Eng. **25**, 1 (2017)
15. Nef, T., Guidali, M., Riener, R.: ARMin III – arm therapy exoskeleton with an ergonomic shoulder actuation. Appl. Bionics Biomech. **6**(2), 127–142 (2009)
16. Khor, K.X., Chin, P.J.H., Rahman, H.A., Yeong, C.F., Narayanan, A.L.T., Su, E.L.M.: Development of reconfigurable rehabilitation robot for post-stroke forearm and wrist training. J. Teknol. **72**(2), 1–5 (2015)
17. Rohrer, B., et al.: Movement smoothness changes during stroke recovery. J. Neurosci. **22**(18), 8297–8304 (2002)

Balance Assessment for Double and Single Leg Stance Using FIBOD Balance System

Kang Xiang Khor[1][(✉)], Che Fai Yeong[1,2], Eileen Lee Ming Su[1],
Hadafi Fitri Mohd Latip[3,4,5], Yvonne Yee Woon Khor[3,4,5], Sook Chin Chan[6],
Phei Ming Chern[7], Mei Lian Leow[7], Najib bin Abdullah[1],
Muhammad Farhan bin Mustar[1], and Muhammad Nurhakim bin Abdul Halim[8]

[1] School of Electrical Engineering, Faculty of Engineering, Universiti Teknologi Malaysia
(UTM), 81300 Skudai, Johor, Malaysia
xiangkk@gmail.com, cfyeong@utm.my
[2] Center of Artificial Intelligence and Robotics, UTM, 54100 Kuala Lumpur, Malaysia
[3] School of Biomedical Engineering and Health Science, Faculty of Engineering, UTM, 81310
Skudai, Johor, Malaysia
[4] Sports Innovation and Technology Centre, UTM, 81300 Skudai, Johor, Malaysia
[5] Institute of Human Centered Engineering (iHumEn), UTM, 81310 Skudai, Johor, Malaysia
[6] Faculty of Health and Sport Sciences (FHSS), MAHSA University, 42610 Jenjarom, Selangor,
Malaysia
[7] Clinical Research Centre, Cheras Rehabilitation Hospital, 56000 Kuala Lumpur, Malaysia
[8] Faculty of Computer and Mathematical Sciences, UiTM, 85000 Segamat, Malaysia

Abstract. Physical balance is important to support human motion for almost all activities of daily living such as standing, sitting, cooking, housework or shopping. However, balance tends to drop as human grow older due to the loss of muscle. FIBOD balance system (FBS) is a balance system designed to be portable and easy to use. This study investigates the FBS balance measures with 17 healthy subjects. Results show significant differences in double-leg overall stability index (OSI) and medial-lateral stability index (MLSI) ($p = 0.01$); double-leg and dominant leg MLSI ($p < 0.001$); double-leg and non-dominant leg MLSI ($p < 0.001$); dominant leg OSI and non-dominant MLSI ($p = 0.02$); double-leg and dominant leg sway velocity ($p = 0.02$) and double-leg and non-dominant leg sway velocity ($p < 0.001$). The results were consistent with existing balance measure from other study. This study also found MLSI and sway velocity to be better features as balance indicator because they were more sensitive in detecting differences between double-leg stance against single-leg stance (dominant or non-dominant leg). Results from this study indicated that the portable FBS is a feasible alternative balance assessment system.

Keywords: Balance board · Balance assessment · Instrumented wobble board

1 Introduction

All activities of daily living, such as standing, sitting, cooking, housework or shopping require physical balance to support the human motion [1, 2]. However, balance tends to

© Springer Nature Switzerland AG 2021
F. Ibrahim et al. (Eds.): ICIBEL 2019, IFMBE Proceedings 81, pp. 103–110, 2021.
https://doi.org/10.1007/978-3-030-65092-6_12

deteriorate with age due to the loss of muscle [3]. Thus, balance assessment is important to evaluate a person's balancing capability from time to time [4]. Several systems had been used to assess human balance such as force plates, Biodex balance system (BBS) and APDM balance sensor. Force plate is used to measure static balance by determining the movement of the center of pressure (COP) [5]. APDM determines the postural sway area while in standing position using a wearable sensor [6]. BBS use a circular moving platform to measure the balance using the anterior-posterior (AP) and medial-lateral (ML) axes simultaneously [7]. It allows balance measurement at dynamic conditions and the determination of ankle joint movement information at the same time[8]. However, BBS is designed to be targeted for institutional usage with more budget and space.

FIBOD balance system (FBS) as shown in the Fig. 1 is a balance system designed to be portable and easy to use [9, 10]. It mimics the widely used wobble board design with a build-in motion sensor for collection of balance performance [11–14]. Fig. 2 shows the variation different posture training and assessment by using FBS. FBS provide five balance measures in the software. The balance measures are medial-lateral stability index (MLSI), anterior-posterior stability index (APSI), overall stability index (OSI), sway velocity, balance zone [7]. The stability index is deviation of the position from the center, the lower the value the higher the stability. Sway velocity is the mean speed, the higher the value the lower the stability. The goal of this study is to determine the performance of double and single leg stance by using FBS balance measures.

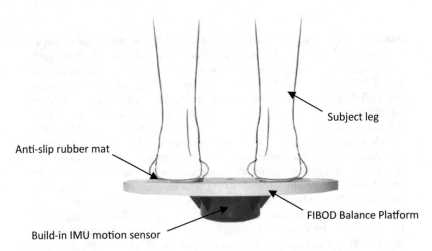

Fig. 1. FIBOD platform overview with double leg standing illustration.

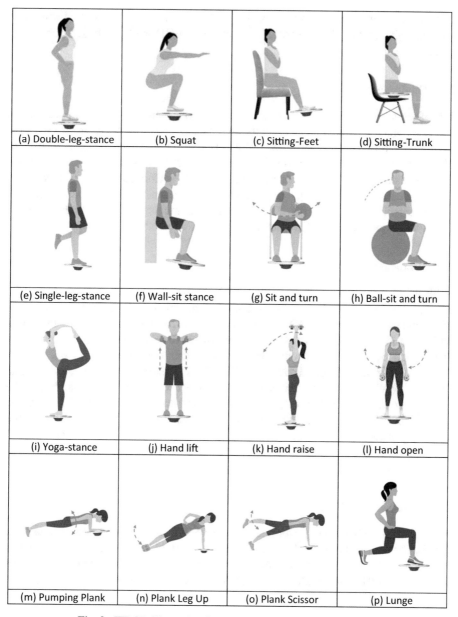

Fig. 2. FIBOD illustration for different training and assessment.

2 Methods

2.1 Subjects

Seventeen healthy subjects (11 males, 6 females, age $= 22.35 \pm 2.69$ years; weight $= 61.84 \pm 15.27$ kg; height $= 165.56 \pm 8.69$ cm, BMI $= 22.39 \pm 4.18$) with no intake of sedatives or alcohol within the past 48 h volunteered and gave informed consent to participate in the study. They were able to stand on FIBOD safely, without reporting any pain.

2.2 Equipment

FIBOD is used in this study, it is a compact, portable and wireless balance system that is designed for training and quantifying balance movement. Multiple customizable training program is provided to allow various exercise for targeted movement. It provides objective assessment to assess body balance and ankle stability and can be incorporated into the training and assessment program for sport performance, rehabilitation, and general wellness services [10]. Study shows the motion sensor data accuracy is ±0.04% and repeatability is ±0.06° [9]. FIBOD device communicates with a Android device through Bluetooth connectivity with data sampling rate of 20 Hz.

2.3 Protocol

Subject was instructed to stand on FIBOD using two legs at specified leg position (refer Fig. 2a). The first trial was a familiarization session, which consisted of maximum 120 s of practice standing on FIBOD. The subject was given 30 s' break before evaluation took place. During evaluation, subject was instructed to stand on FIBOD using two legs at specified leg position for evaluation. Evaluation data was collected by FBS software for 10 s while the subject balanced the FIBOD as horizontal as possible with visual feedback provided at the monitor screen. The subject was given 15 s' break before the next trial and the trial was repeated three times. After completion of 3 double leg trials, subject would rest for 10 min. Next, the subject was asked to balance the FIBOD using single-leg (refer Fig. 2e). Similarly, the trial would be repeated 3 times each with left and right leg respectively. Subjects were not allowed to use support aid throughout trial and data collection period.

2.4 Statistical Analysis

All statistical analysis was performed using the SPSS v20 statistical analysis package (IBM). The normality of the data was determined using Shapiro-Wilk test and all data was found to be of normal distribution. Statistical significance test between the groups was done using the t-test with $\alpha < 0.05$ indicating statistical significance.

3 Result

Table 1 presented the result of balance measures for double-leg, left-leg and right-leg stance test. The OSI mean for double-leg, left- and right-leg stance is 5.11 ± 3.01, 4.67 ± 2.21 and 4.55 ± 2.99 respectively. Sway velocity of left leg is the highest at 12.06 ± 5.97°/s. The largest inner zone was from right-leg stance at 78.72 ± 24.04%. The highest middle zone was from left leg stance at 20.17 ± 17.10% and the highest outer zone was 6.75 ± 12.46% from double leg stance. The highest fall percentage is from double

Table 1. Balance measures of double-leg, left-leg and right-leg stance test

No.	Balance measures	Double-leg stance test (Mean ± SD)	Left-leg stance test (Mean ± SD)	Right-leg stance test (Mean ± SD)
1	OSI	5.11 ± 3.01	4.67 ± 2.21	4.55 ± 2.99
2	APSI	4.12 ± 2.54	3.82 ± 2.03	3.69 ± 2.68
3	MLSI	2.87 ± 1.75	2.53 ± 1.09	2.60 ± 1.54
4	SV (°/s)	5.99 ± 2.78	12.06 ± 5.97	9.77 ± 5.21
5	IZ (%)	76.28 ± 21.48	77.24 ± 21.47	78.72 ± 24.04
6	MZ (%)	18.01 ± 12.24	20.17 ± 17.10	17.47 ± 16.11
7	OZ (%)	6.75 ± 12.46	4.17 ± 5.99	5.59 ± 13.87
8	FI (%)	21.84 ± 13.20	20.16 ± 10.87	18.17 ± 12.82

OSI = Overall Stability Index, APSI = Anterior-Posterior Stability Index, MLSI = Medial-Lateral Stability Index, SV = Sway Velocity, IZ = Inner zone percentage, MZ = middle zone percentage, OZ = outer zone percentage, FI = fall indication percentage.

Table 2. Comparison of stability index between double, dominant and non-dominant leg

No	Stability index 1	Stability index 2	Mean ± SD 1	Mean ± SD 2	$P < 0.05$*
1	DL-OSI	DL-APSI	5.11 ± 3.01	4.12 ± 2.54	0.31
2	DL-OSI	DL-MLSI	5.11 ± 3.01	2.87 ± 1.75	**0.01***
3	DL-OSI	DO-OSI	5.11 ± 3.01	4.40 ± 2.98	0.49
4	DL-OSI	DO-APSI	5.11 ± 3.01	3.61 ± 2.70	0.14
5	DL-OSI	DO-MLSI	5.11 ± 3.01	2.46 ± 1.43	**< 0.01***
6	DL-OSI	ND-OSI	5.11 ± 3.01	4.87 ± 2.21	0.79
7	DL-OSI	ND-APSI	5.11 ± 3.01	3.92 ± 2.00	0.18
8	DL-OSI	ND-MLSI	5.11 ± 3.01	2.73 ± 1.25	**< 0.01***
9	DO-OSI	DO-APSI	4.40 ± 2.98	3.61 ± 2.70	0.42
10	DO-OSI	DO-MLSI	4.40 ± 2.98	2.46 ± 1.43	**0.02***
11	DO-OSI	ND-OSI	4.40 ± 2.98	4.87 ± 2.21	0.60
12	DO-APSI	ND-APSI	3.61 ± 2.70	3.92 ± 2.00	0.71
13	DO-MLSI	ND-MLSI	2.46 ± 1.43	2.73 ± 1.25	0.56
14	DL-SV	DO-SV	5.99 ± 2.78	9.64 ± 5.27	**0.02***
15	DL-SV	ND-SV	5.99 ± 2.78	11.63 ± 6.26	**< 0.01***
16	DO-SV	ND-SV	9.64 ± 5.27	11.63 ± 6.26	0.32

OSI = Overall Stability Index, APSI = Anterior-Posterior Stability Index, MLSI = Medial-Lateral Stability Index, SV = Sway Velocity, DL = Double-leg Stance Test, DO = Dominant-leg Stance Test, ND = Non-Dominant-leg Stance Test.
* = $p < 0.05$, ** = $p < 0.01$

leg stance at 21.84 ± 13.20%. Table 2 shows the comparison of stability index between double, dominant and non-dominant leg. Results show significant differences between double-leg OSI and MLSI (p = 0.01); double-leg and dominant leg MLSI (p < .001); double-leg and non-dominant leg MLSI (p < .001); dominant leg OSI and non-dominant MLSI (p = 0.02); double-leg and dominant leg sway velocity (p = 0.02) and double-leg and non-dominant leg sway velocity (p < .001).

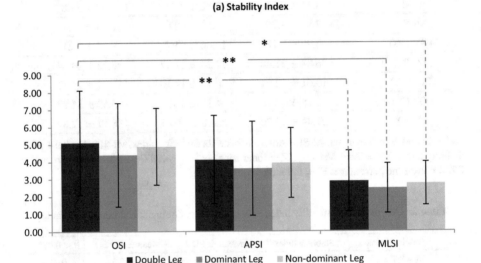

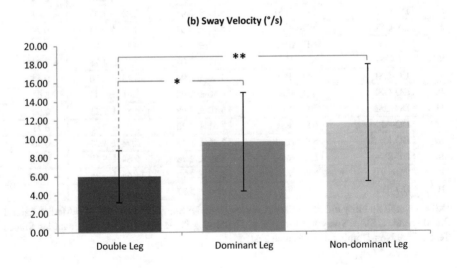

Fig. 3. Comparison of double leg, dominant and non-dominant leg balance measures: (a) Stability index and (b) Sway velocity.

Figure 3 shows the comparison of double leg, dominant and non-dominant leg balance measures. Results show double leg stance OSI was significantly different from double, dominant and non-dominant leg MLSI. Double leg sway velocity shows significant difference compared to dominant and non-dominant leg.

4 Discussion

This section discussed the relationships between double, dominant, non-dominant, left and right leg stance in balance measurement. Sway velocity of left leg recorded the highest average value, possibly because most subjects were right leg dominant and were unstable when performing using their non-dominant leg. The largest inner zone percentage recorded for right leg stance also showed the characteristic as expected from a majority right leg dominant population. The highest outer zone percentage from double leg stance was due to the body coordination and larger range of movement when both legs were standing on the board. The balance measures recorded for APSI tends to be higher than MLSI. This is due to the nature of ankle anatomy, in which anterior-posterior (AP) has wider range of movement compared to medial-lateral (ML) direction. The smaller values mean ML instabilities could be overlooked if only OSI was used for balance assessment. This is because OSI is the combination of AP and ML motion and APSI tends to be more dominant in OSI. Based on our findings, MLSI, APSI and sway velocity may best be used separately as MLSI and sway velocity are more sensitive in detecting differences between 2 legs against dominant or non-dominant leg. This may be important for clinical investigation when determining the instability of the leg and for clinical evaluation of leg balancing. The limitations of this study included the subject group's heterogeneity. Several subjects have indicated previous mild muscle injuries, of which they have recovered, while some are trained school athletes, which may have caused differences in balance performance compared to normal population.

5 Conclusion

From this study, it was found that MLSI and sway velocity recorded significant differences between double leg stance with single leg stance while OSI and APSI did not show statistical differences between the two stances. Hence, MLSI and sway velocity may be better features for stability indicator in clinical assessment. The balance measures of OSI, MLSI, and APSI from this study were consistent with results reported in previous Biodex Balance System study, making the portable FIBOD Balance System a feasible alternative for high performance balance assessment.

Acknowledgement. The authors would like to express their gratitude to National Stroke Association of Malaysia (NASAM), MAHSA University, Clinical Research Center Cheras Rehabilitation Hospital, Ministry of Education (MOE), Malaysia and Biofit Technologies & Services for the contribution to the work. This work is supported by the Universiti Teknologi Malaysia research grant [04H66, 06H86, 04G42, 16H47], and Collaborative Research in Engineering, Science and Teknologi Center (CREST) R&D grant [P37C2-13].

References

1. Judge, J.: Balance training to maintain mobility and prevent disability. Am. J. Prev. Med. **25**(3), 150–156 (2003)
2. Judge, J.O., Schechtman, K., Cress, E., Group, F.: The relationship between physical performance measures and independence in instrumental activities of daily living. J. Am. Geriatr. Soc. **44**(11), 1332–1341 (1996)
3. Kallman, D.A., Plato, C.C., Tobin, J.D.: The role of muscle loss in the age-related decline of grip strength: cross-sectional and longitudinal perspectives. J. Gerontol. **45**(3), M82–M88 (1990)
4. Mancini, M., Horak, F.B.: The relevance of clinical balance assessment tools to differentiate balance deficits. Eur. J. Phys. Rehabil. Med. **46**(2), 239–248 (2010)
5. Karlsson, A., Frykberg, G.: Correlations between force plate measures for assessment of balance. Clin. Biomech. **15**(5), 365–369 (2000)
6. Laurie King, M.M.: Mobility lab to assess balance and gait with synchronized body-worn sensors. J. Bioeng. Biomed. Sci. 1–5 (2013)
7. Arnold, B.L., Schmitz, R.J.: Examination of balance measures produced by the biodex stability system. J. Athl. Train. **33**(4), 323–327 (1998)
8. Pereira, H.M., de Campos, T.F., Santos, M.B., Cardoso, J.R., de Camargo Garcia, M., Cohen, M.: Influence of knee position on the postural stability index registered by the Biodex Stability System. Gait Posture **28**(4), 668–672 (2008)
9. Xiang, K.K., bin Mustar, M.F., bin Abdullah, N., Fai, Y.C., bin Darsim, M.N., Ming, E. S.L.: Development of InnovaBoard: an interactive balance board for balancing training and ankle rehabilitation. In: 2016 IEEE International Symposium on Robotics and Intelligent Sensors (IRIS), pp. 128–133 (2016)
10. Khor, K.X., et al.: Smart balance board to improve balance and reduce fall risk: pilot study. In: IFMBE Proceedings, vol. 67 (2018)
11. Park, T.-J.: The effects of wobble board training on the eyes open and closed static balance ability of adolescents with down syndrome. J. Phys. Ther. Sci. **26**(4), 625–627 (2014)
12. Waddington, G., Adams, R., Jones, A.: Wobble board (ankle disc) training effects on the discrimination of inversion movements. Aust. J. Physiother. **45**(2), 95–101 (1999)
13. Clark, V.M., Burden, A.M.: A 4-week wobble board exercise programme improved muscle onset latency and perceived stability in individuals with a functionally unstable ankle. Phys. Ther. Sport **6**(4), 181–187 (2005)
14. Wester, J.U., Jespersen, S.M., Nielsen, K.D., Neumann, L.: Wobble board training after partial sprains of the lateral ligaments of the ankle: a prospective randomized study. J. Orthop. Sport. Phys. Ther. **23**(5), 332–336 (1996)

Ergonomic Risks on Smartphone Addiction Among University Students

N. Roslizawati$^{(\boxtimes)}$ and I. Isyan Farahin

Physiotherapy Program School of Health Sciences, KPJ Healthcare University College,
Nilai, Malaysia
ucn.roslizawati@kpjuc.edu.my

Abstract. Excessive smartphone usage caused musculoskeletal health problems. However, there is no clear understanding on how smartphone addiction impaired health. Posture adoption and its risk while using smartphone might contribute towards health problem which not yet been determined especially among university students who also using smartphone for learning activities. Therefore, this study aims at determine ergonomic risk and physical exposures on smartphone usage among university students. A cross-sectional study was conducted at a Private University in Nilai. A total of 310 students aged between 18 to 30 (21 ± 2.17) years old who are using smartphone were participated in this study. Postural analysis tool using Rapid Upper Limb Assessment (RULA) were used to determine ergonomic risk and physical exposures. Distribution of ergonomics risk and its exposures with smartphone usage was analysed by using descriptive analysis. Study has showed that university students were addicted to their smartphone with high daily usage for 12 h per day since 6–7 years ago. They were used smartphone for social media (99%) and games (75.2%). Smartphone helps students to be more socialize (71%). Students has high usage of smartphone which longer than they had intended (61%) causing lack of adequate sleep (68%) and tiredness (82.8%). Students were also found to have experienced with awkward body and static body posture while using smartphone. Students were also using smartphone both in standing and sitting. They hold and use smartphone with awkward hand grip and awkward hand movement, with high repetition at high speed. Most of them prefer to use smartphone with vibration mode. RULA score while using smartphone showed that university students were experienced with moderate risk at upper arm and wrist (4.77 ± 0.86) which require changing the pattern of usage soon as and it should be taken into high consideration. Whereas, RULA score for neck, trunk and leg was at 4 (4.13 ± 1.10) require them to be investigated further. The grand total of RULA score showed that ergonomic risk at 4.77 ± 1.13 (risk level range: 5–6), indicate that the student's postures while using smartphone need to be investigated further and require to change soon. They are require an intervention of ergonomic awareness for them to change the posture adopted while using smartphone as soon as possible. Therefore, this study concluded that university students were addicted to smartphone which has increase physical exposures such as awkward posture, static posture, awkward hand grip and movement, high speed, repetitive and vibration at hand which subsequently affect their ergonomic risk. The finding was significant in improving awareness on posture while using smartphone. Ergonomic intervention should incorporate with consultation on posture correction and awareness related to risk of smartphone addiction.

F. Ibrahim et al. (Eds.): ICIBEL 2019, IFMBE Proceedings 81, pp. 111–117, 2021.
https://doi.org/10.1007/978-3-030-65092-6_13

Keywords: Smartphone addiction · Ergonomic risk · University students

1 Introduction

Occupational discomfort due to work-relatedness disorder is a multifactorial problem. There are conflicting evidences with regards to posture as a risk factor, with studies reporting sitting as a major contributing factor but no conclusive evidence of increased risk [1]. There are more consensuses that static postures exacerbate MSD but how the static posture during smart phone usage could effect on the risk of MSDs is not well known.

Contribution of smartphone usage and its effects on neck and shoulder pain among in Malaysia has been determined [2]. However, there is no pre-determined physical exposure and ergonomic risk on posture adopted while using smart phone. Furthermore, there is no clear understanding on relationship between phone addiction and its among young adults in university population. Previous study also has postulated that excessive use of mobile phones caused health problems [3]. Excessive smartphone usage leads to headache (63.3%), memory problems (28.5%) and depression (19.69%). These effects affected by individual posture control. Even when two persons performing similar postures with using smartphone, there may still be some differences in individual postures assumed which may have contributed to some of variations in their physical exposures and ergonomic risks. Besides the proposed anticipatory feed-forward motor control mechanism, the postural habits of the individuals which are likely to be interdependent to movements control which influenced by muscle fatigue, and discomfort following a static low level activity [4]. Thus, the smartphone usage and its influence of postural control and contribution toward ergonomic risk are fundamental to be carried out.

Therefore, this study aims at investigating the smartphone usage and ergonomic risk among university students. The finding of this study would enhance more understanding on health background among students in related to their smartphone usage. Identifying the risk factors into ergonomic awareness is fundamental to overcome symptoms and the cause root of musculoskeletal disorders among students which are still lacking. In Malaysia, lack of ergonomic awareness is a great concern that contributes towards work-related musculoskeletal complains. Malaysian global legislative effort is needed to enhance the importance of ergonomic awareness to minimize complains of musculoskeletal disorders.

Thus, evidence-based information regarding sources of work-related stress such as ergonomic risk and physical exposure would be useful to provide baseline reference in designing the proper safety and health guidelines in Malaysian, which are still lacking and become scope of interest in this study.

2 Methodology

A cross-sectional study was conducted among 311 students at a Private University College in Nilai who aged ranged between 18 to 27 years old (20.85 ± 1.94). Students were used smartphone minimum 6 months were recruited voluntarily through a convenience sampling. The total sample size of participants representing the population which was determined using Krejeic & Morgan table [5]. Ethical approval has been obtained from Institutional Ethical Board prior for this study to be conducted. Subjects were volunteers and human right was protected. This study has investigated ergonomic risk during smartphone usage by using Rapid Upper Limb Assessment (RULA) [6]. The postural analysis tool was reliable to be used in assessing biomechanical and postural loading on work-related disorders, particularly in the neck, trunk and the upper limb. Participant's posture while using mobile phone has been observed and assessed without any instruction which not to distract their concentration.

Assessment of RULA involve 3 steps: scoring of working posture for each body part, grouping the body part posture and development of grand score. A score from 1 indicates the most neutral position to range of 4 maximum score which indicates the worst position for each body part. Score A was presented the combined individual scores for shoulder, elbow and wrist and score B is calculated from neck, trunk and legs. Muscle use and force exerted attributing a score of 1 and 0 respectively which represented the both groups performed static posture and no adding load. These score are added to each score of A and B to obtain score C and D. The combination of scores C and D determined the 'grand score' which reflects the postural and musculoskeletal load. The total grand scores indicate work posture and load are: acceptable (score 1 or 2), require investigate further (score 3 or 4), to investigate further and change soon (score 5 and 6) or to investigate and change immediately (score 7). The assessment was carried out using worksheet (Fig. 1).

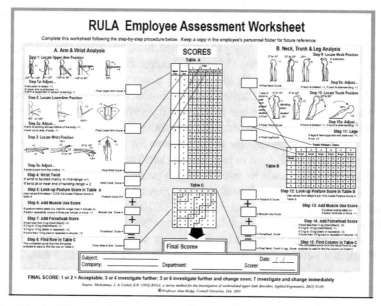

Fig. 1. RULA worksheet. Source: McAtamney, L. & Corlett, E.N. (1993)

Ergonomic exposures which might influence by smartphone usage was also investigated such awkward body posture, static body posture, awkward grip, awkward hand movement, repetitive task, sitting, standing and usage of vibration. They were asked to rate the frequency of exposures during smartphone usage on a 5-likert scale ranging from 0 = never (does not occur at all), 1 = occasional (1–2 times per day), 2 = often (3–5 times per day) and 3 = always (more than 5 times per day or continuously). Descriptive analysis has explained physical exposures and ergonomic risk by using frequency distribution. Frequency table was used to present analysis of findings.

3 Results

Study has showed that university students were addicted to their smartphone with high daily usage for 12 h per day since 6–7 years ago. They were used smartphone with right hand (93%) for social media (99%) and games (75.2%). Smartphone helps students to be more socialize (71%). Students has high usage of smartphone which longer than they had intended (61%) causing lack of adequate sleep (68%) and tiredness (82.8%).

This study have showed that students were experienced awkward body and static body posture occasionally while using smartphone. When holding smartphone for usage, they were occasionally tend to performed hand grip and hand movement awkwardly. Smartphone usage also not causing them to do lifting, pushing and pulling. However, most of them were experienced repetitive task and working in high speed when use smartphone. Students were also using smartphone both in standing and sitting. Most of them prefer to use vibrates mode of smartphone. Table 2 reported frequency of ergonomic exposures experiences by students with smartphone usage.

Ergonomic risk was assessed by using RULA and found the risk at 4.77 ± 0.86 (risk level range: 5–6) for score A indicated that upper arm and wrist while using smartphone experienced with moderate risk. Study has revealed that while subjects using smartphone, their upper arm were position at +45° to 90° shoulder flexion, upper arm abducted and shoulder moves repeatedly. While lower arm position were at elbow 90° flexion and frequent across arm adduct and wrist flexion/extension about 15° with combination of radial deviation, ulnar deviation and twisting of the wrist. The actions were repeatedly occur 4 times per min and more thus this increasing the scores of the arm and wrist analysis. Therefore, this finding has showed a need for them to be investigated further and awareness has to be address to manage the risk. They require changing the pattern of usage soon as and it should be taken into high consideration.

Whereas, Score B which reflected risk experienced by neck, trunk and leg position while using smartphone were showed at 4.13 ± 1.10 (risk level range: 3–4), indicated neck, trunk and leg position among subjects were at low risk. Means, subjects were using smartphone with neck at 20° of flexion with the trunk flexion and rotation repeatedly at 0° to 20° and this posture were repeatedly done in cycle more than 4 min. They were required to be investigated further but ergonomics intervention is not at urge.

The grand score which considered risks at score A and B has showed that at 4.77 ± 1.13 (risk level range: 5–6) indicated that student postures while using smartphone need to be investigated and some changes are required immediately. Students were at moderate risk for both upper limb and lower limb contributions. They are require an intervention of ergonomic awareness for them to change the pattern as soon as possible. Frequency distribution also showed that most of students found at medium risk levels (RULA score 5–6) require further investigation and need to change soon (48%). Whereas a total of 45.9% of students were experienced low risk (RULA score 3–4) which require to be investigated further. However, less students who had experienced with high risk (RULA score 7) while using smartphone (5.8%) (Table 1).

Table 1. Ergonomic risk by RULA (Grand Score) experienced among university students while using smartphones

RULA level	0	1	2	3
RULA Score	1-2	3-4	5-6	7
Risk Level	Negligible	Low	Medium	High
Require Action	Acceptable	Investigate further	Investigate further and change soon	Investigate and change immediately
Frequency of students (%)	–	45.9	48.3	5.8

Table 2. Ergonomic exposures experienced by students with smartphone usage.

Ergonomic exposures	Frequency (%)			
	Never	Occasional	Often	Always
Awkward body	16.2	41.3	30.4	12.2
Static body	22.4	39.3	27.4	10.9
Awkward grip	25.4	38.9	21.8	13.9
Awkward hand	32	36	19.5	12.5
Repetitive task	20.1	33	28.7	18.2
Working high speed	19.5	35	29.7	15.5
Standing	12.2	29	32.3	26.4
Sitting	9.2	8.3	8.3	50.2
Vibrates tools	22.8	27.1	24.1	26.1

4   Discussion

The frequency of phone usage daily among students was high which reported for 12 h per day since 6–7 years of usage which more than frequency of smartphone usage by university students of Saudi Arabia which reported with 27.2% of student spent more than 8 h per day using their smartphone and 75% of them used at least 4 applications per day [7]. This study showed that students were addicted to their smartphone. The finding has been justified that the time of smartphone usage and addiction severity was found to be correlated [8]. The more of individual spent with smartphone, the more they tend to be smartphone addicted. The amount of usage influences the addiction among smartphone users.

Addiction of smartphone affected daily living activities. Increase severity of smartphone addiction exposed university students to experience with awkward body, awkward hand and repetitive task causing them to have lack of adequate sleep and felt tired. Similarly, university students in Saudi Arabia had also decrease sleeping hours and experienced a lack of energy the next day as a results of smartphone addiction [9]. Smartphone addiction has correlated with poor sleep quality and leads to depression and anxiety [10].

Previous study has suggested on difference sleep duration in comparing students who used smartphone with old version or latest technology advance application [10]. Sleeps duration of students who use latest technology advance application mobile phone were 5.43 h at night time and 7.2 h per day. Whereas, average sleeps duration of students, who used old version of the mobile phone with fewer applications were 6.53 h per night and 8.3 h per day. Therefore, students who use latest technology which can access with more applications are more addicted to their smartphones. The findings was similar with found among students in Turkey which reported over 50% of students were used smartphone for WhatsApp, Instagram, YouTube, Facebook and Snapchat were more addicted to their smartphones. Students in Turkey were also reported preferably using smartphone for WhatsApp, Instagram, YouTube, Facebook and Snapchat [11].

The findings justify that university students has experienced high ergonomic risk due to smartphone addiction. Most of them score of high risk which indicates further investigations and change is needed. The finding was similar with students of Rural Medical College in India who adopted awkward postures when using smartphones and they also had high ergonomic risk [12]. Previous studies also supported that prolong usage of smartphone and smartphone addiction cause higher ergonomic risk among students in Filipina [13] and Taiwan [14]. They also reported having experience with more depressive symptoms, higher positive outcome expectancy of internet use, higher Internet usage time, lower refusal self-efficacy of internet use, higher impulsivity, lower satisfaction with academic performance and insecurity.

5   Conclusion

This study has determined smartphone usage and its influence on ergonomic risk experience by student. University students were addicted to smartphone which exposed them to have higher ergonomic risk. The finding was significant in improving awareness on posture while using smartphone. Ergonomic intervention should incorporate with consultation on posture correction and awareness related to smartphone usage. Postural correction while using smartphone should be encounter to prevent risk of neck and upper extremity pain among young adult. Thus, finding from this study is benefited in providing evidence-based information towards efficacy of ergonomic posture awareness aims at musculoskeletal health.

Acknowledgement. Authors would like to gratefully thanks to School of Health Sciences, KPJ Healthcare University College for highly support and respondents who volunteered to participate in this study.

References

1. Weevers, H.A., van der Beek, A.J., Anema, J.R., van der Wal, G., Mechelen, W.V.: Work-related disease in general practice: a systemic review. ProQuest Health Med. Complete **22**(2), 197 (2005)
2. Kalirathinam, D., Manoharlal, M.A., Mei, C., Ling, C.K., Sheng, T.W., Jerome, A., Rao, U.M.: Association between the usage of smartphone as the risk factor for the prevalence of upper extremity and neck symptoms among university students: a cross-sectional survey based study. Res. J. Pharm. Technol. **10**(4), 1184 (2017)
3. AlZarea, B.K., Patil, S.R.: Mobile phone head and neck pain syndrome: proposal of a new entity. Headache **251**, 63–3 (2015)
4. Madeleine, P.: On Functional motor adaptations: from the quantification of motor strategies to the prevention of musculoskeletal disorders in the neck-shoulder region. Acta Physiol. **199**, 1–46 (2010)
5. Krejcie, R.V., Morgan, D.W.: Determining sample size for research activities. Educ. Psychol. Meas. **30**, 607–610 (1970)
6. Mc Atamney L., Corlett E.N.: RULA: a survey method for the investigation of work-related upper limb disorders. Appl. Ergon. **24**(2), 91–99 (1993)
7. Alosaimi, F., Alyahya, H., Alshahwan, H., Mahyijari, N.A., Shaik, S.: Smartphone addiction among university students in Riyadh. Saudi Arabia. Saudi Med. J. **37**(6), 675–683 (2016)
8. Hwang, K.H., Yoo, Y.S., Cho, O.H.: Smartphone overuse and upper extremity pain, anxiety, depression, and interpersonal relationships among college students. J. Korea Contents Assoc. **12**(10), 365–375 (2012)
9. Chen, B., Liu, F., Ding, S., Ying, X., Wang, L., Wen, Y.: Gender differences in factors associated with smartphone addiction: a cross-sectional study among medical college students. BMC Psychiatry **17**(1), 341 (2017)
10. Bhatti, U., Rani, K., Memon, M.Q., Wali, H.: Effects of advanced cell phone technology on the duration of sleep. New York Sci. J. **8**, 86–88 (2015)
11. Yasemin S., Omer OSmartphone addiction and the use of social media among university students. Mediterr. J. Humanit. **7**, 367–377 (2017)
12. Ravija, G., Deepali, H.: Correlation Of ergonomic risks and upper extremity musculoskeletal disorders among smartphone user medical students. Int. J. Med. Sci. Diagn. Res. **3**(3), 17–22 (2019)
13. Jannie, L.C., John, B.C., Adam, H.D., John, R.M., Ryan, V., Lizbeth, M.: Ergonomic risk assessment for the prolonged usage of Smartphones on students. Adv. Phys. Ergon. Human Factors (2019). https://doi.org/10.1007/978-3-319-94484-5_16
14. Lin, M.P., Ko, H.C., Wu, J.Y.W.: Prevalence and psychosocial risk factors associated with Internet addiction in a nationally representative sample of college students in Taiwan. Cyberpsychology, Behav. Soc. Networking **14**(12), 741–746 (2011)

Theme: Biosensing and Life Sciences

Entropy-Based EEG Markers for Gender Identification of Vascular Dementia Patients

Noor Kamal Al-Qazzaz[1,2]($\boxtimes$), Sawal Hamid Md Ali[1], and Siti Anom Ahmad[3,4]

[1] Department of Electrical, Electronic and Systems Engineering, Faculty of Engineering and Built Environment, Universiti Kebangsaan Malaysia, UKM, 43600 Bangi, Selangor, Malaysia
noorbmemsc@gmail.com
[2] Department of Biomedical Engineering, Al-Khwarizmi College of Engineering, University of Baghdad, Baghdad 47146, Iraq
[3] Department of Electrical and Electronic Engineering Faculty of Engineering, Universiti Putra Malaysia, UPM, 43400 Serdang, Selangor, Malaysia
[4] Malaysian Research Institute of Ageing (MyAgeing), Universiti Putra Malaysia, 43400 Serdang, Selangor, Malaysia

Abstract. The efforts in this study were being made to understand how gender differences contribute to identifying the early signs of cognitive impairment that were lead to severe dementia. The electroencephalogram (EEG) of 5 patients with vascular dementia (VD), 15 stroke-related mild cognitive impairment (S_MCI) patients, and 15 healthy control (HC) subjects during a working memory task (WMT). To do so, Savitzky–Golay (SG) filter was applied in the first stage as a preprocessing method for the seek of EEG signals smoothing and artifacts removal. In the second stage, four different entropies were extracted from the denoised EEG signals to test the hypothesis of reducing the complexity in both VD and S_MCI in comparison with HC these are spectral entropy (*SpecEn*), fuzzy entropy (*FuzEn*), tsallis entropy (*TsEn*) and improved permutation entropy (*impe*). In the next step, statistical analysis has been conducted by using multivariate analysis of variance (MANOVA) to assess the gender differences over the brain regions for S_MCI and dementia patients compared with HC subjects. Results show that the entropy-based EEG analyses may provide a simple method with a cost-effective way to identify and quantify the severity of dementia patients. In conclusion, increased dementia severity was associated with decreased entropy-based features complexity. Thus, EEG could be the key to report interesting information for differentiation the EEG background activity in female and male of patients with VD and S_MCI to help medical doctors to identify gender differences effects on dementia survivors.

Keywords: Vascular dementia · Electroencephalogram savitzky–golay · Entropy · Multivariate analysis of variance

1 Introduction

Vascular dementia (VD) is considered as the major health problems following stroke onset in the elderly population. Most of the stroke survivors' were prone to get dementia

© Springer Nature Switzerland AG 2021
F. Ibrahim et al. (Eds.): ICIBEL 2019, IFMBE Proceedings 81, pp. 121–128, 2021.
https://doi.org/10.1007/978-3-030-65092-6_14

by the first year of stroke diagnosis. Therefore, VD can be defined as the progressive impairment in memory that ends up with a decline in the patient activity of daily living [1]. The prodromal stage of VD dementia is known as mild cognitive impairment (MCI) due to a stroke which characterized by a mild decline in mental thinking for 10–15% of them may develop dementia per year, however, some of MCI patients may remain stable [2]. Many risk factors are associated with stroke and dementia, these are the modifiable risk factors including cerebral vascular disease (CVD) such as: hypertension, heart disease, and diabetes mellitus which are the highest factors for stroke and post-stroke dementia (PSD) [3–8], whereas, the non-modifiable risk factors, including age, gender, ethnicity and genetics [1, 9].

Efforts are being made to understand how gender differences contribute to dementia risk and how dementia could be identified early to provide suitable neurofeedback rehabilitation; therefore, different studies have been performed to deserve this issue. Researchers have studied the relationship between dementia and gender, they found that dementia has a higher incidence rate in female compared to male particularly after the eighties [10].

As dementia survivors gradually lose the brain cells and that leads to impairment and dysfunction in attention and working memory [1, 9, 11]. Therefore, an urgent need for widely available low-cost Electroencephalogram (EEG) device that has been used recently as a tool to help diagnose different types of dementia including Alzheimer's disease (AD) and other types of dementia. Numerous EEG literature has been reported that most the dementia abnormalities were associated with slowing the spectral EEG frequency rhythms [12–15]. Other studies have been investigated the effect of dementia on the EEG signals complexity using entropies. In general, dementia patients showed reduced the EEG complexity compared to the control subjects [16, 17].

In this study, the effects of two prominent risk factors for VD and S_MCI were investigated, stroke as a CVD (modifiable risk factor) and gender (non- modifiable risk factor) and these risk factors were eventually leads to the development of PSD after stroke onset. The present study hypothesized that the EEG complexity of VD and S_MCI would could be used to identify gender for the patients whose suffer from cognitive impairment and memory dysfunction compare to HC normal subjects.

This study investigates the changes in the complexity and the dynamics of EEG signals for dementia patients that had cognitive and behavioral dysfunction in memory after a stroke diagnosis. Spectral entropy (*SpecEn*), fuzzy entropy (*FuzEn*), tsallis entropy (*TsEn*) and improved permutation entropy (*impe*) were investigated and extracted from every EEG channel to evaluate the effect of gender differences for S_MCI and VD patients. Therefore, it is important to develop entropy indices based on EEG background that are sensitive to the activity differences in both female and male of patients with VD and S_MCI compared to HC.

2 Methods and Materials

2.1 Methods

In order to identify weather the gender has an influence on developing dementia, EEG signals of dementia patients' will be used. Four types of entropies were extracted to illustrate the gender effects on the dementia at the diagnosis and the changes after dementia onset. EEG dataset need a successive signal processing and analysis stages (Fig. 1).

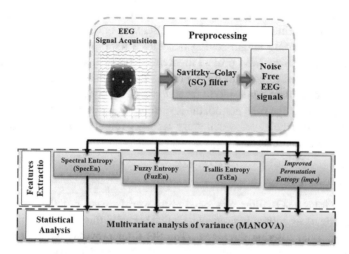

Fig. 1. The block diagram of the proposed method.

2.2 Participants

This study investigates outcomes from the examination of an EEG dataset of 35 patients. The pattern populace used to be recruited from Malyasia's Pusat Perubatan Universiti Kebangsaan (PPUKM) stroke unit, in addition to the institution's neurology clinic. The EEG dataset was once investigated for fifteen healthful manage topics (seven male and eight female, aged 60.06 ± 5.21), fifteen stroke-related S_MCI sufferers (five male and ten female, aged 60.26 ± 7.77) and 5 VD sufferers (three male and two female, aged 64.6 ± 4.8). These three categories have been challenge to the following cognitive evaluations: a mini-mental country examination (MMSE) [7]; The MMSE rating and MoCA rating had been (29.6 ± 0.73, 29.06 ± 0.88) respectively for the manage subjects; for the S_MCI, the MMSE rating and MoCA rating have been (20.2 ± 5.63, 16.13 ± 5.97) respectively. Lastly, for the VD patients, the MMSE rating and MoCA rating had been (14.8 ± 1.92, 14.8 ± 1.92) respectively. The investigative methodologies employed in the course of the lookup had obtained prior approval from the PPUKM's Human Ethics Committee, with knowledgeable voluntary consent of all members was once was once bought by signed consent archives.

2.3 EEG Recording Procedure

NicoletOne (v.32) used to be utilised to acquire the 19 EEG channel datasets. These channels had been obtained as follows: FP2, F8, T4, T6, O2, FP1, F7, T3, T5, O1,

F4, C4, P3, F3, C3, P3, Fz, Cz, and Pz. By utilising a single floor electrode in conjunction with a pair of reference electrodes, a referential montage used to be carried out, with the channel configurations based totally upon the 10–20 global framework. Sampling of the Nicolet EEG tool was sampled with 256 Hz sampling frequency, and electrode-skin impedance was once checked to make sure 10 kilo ohms had been no longer exceeded. During the WM task, the EEG was once captured for a timeframe of 60 s, with a recording length setting out with a fixation cue lasting 0.5 s. Subsequently, a simple auditory WM project involving 5 phrases used to be undertaken, the place sufferers wished to commit these phrases to reminiscence for 10 s [1–3]. Each participant was once then requested to recall the phrases concerned in the EEG recording. On completion of the 60-s period, the investigator requested that the contributors of the pattern team open their eyes, when every was once required to recall in order every of the phrases they remembered.

2.4 Preprocessing Stage

A Savitzky–Golay (SG) filter was once employed to easy out the sign with minimal destruction of its authentic traits [4]. Unlike wavelet, this strategy entails the transferring impact after filtering the signal. The SG filter provides the gain of maintaining the points of a time collection along with its relative minima and maxima, which symbolize a especially giant situation referring to to segmentation of a sign such as EEG [5].

The overall performance of an SG filter is usually reliant on two parameters: the polynomial order and the frame size [6]. Consequently, the coefficients of an SG filter have been geared up to $N = Nr + Nl + 1$ points of the EEG signal, the place N describes window size, Nr and Nl respectively signify sign factors in the proper and sign factors in the left of a present day sign factor [5–7]. Therefore, to denoise and easy the EEG dataset, this investigation set, the SG filter parameters to the third order polynomial and a body measurement of fifty one samples [6].

2.5 Feature Extraction

The brain is a complicated structure, consequently to quantify the complexity of the talent alerts and to discover the abnormalities in all the EEGs' signals, 4 entropy-based metrics have been calculated. Spectral evaluation has been performed the use of *SpecEn* to quantify slowing in frequency following VD and S_MCI. Therefore, to estimate the *SpecEn*, the *PSD* was once normalized to a scale from zero to 1 to get normalized *PSD* (*PSD_n*), afterwards, *SpecEn* computed making use of the Shannon's entropy to the PSD_n for frequency vary (0.5 *to* 64 *Hz*) and it is computed as in [8–10].

FuzEn is used to estimate the similarity for EEG indicators [11, 12]. *FuzEn* values would rely on the values of the enter parameters these are the size of the time collection N, m used to determine the length of the sequences, used to decide the size of the sequences, r and n determine the width and gradient of the fuzzy exponential function [12].*TsEn* used to be first delivered with the aid of Havrda and Charvát and examined in depth with the aid of Daróczy [13, 14]. This entropy measure differs from the popular Boltzman–Gibbs–Shannon entropy measure, the Boltzman–Gibbs–Shannon measure was once generalized to a crew of measures that are no longer always extensive. Instead, they can be subadditive or superadditive [15]. *TsEn* with parameter $q = 1$ have been used. A generalised measure of *TsEn* can be estimated as in [15].

The thought of impe is based totally on the measure of the relative frequencies of distinct motifs. impe additionally affords an alternate way of measuring similarity amongst patterns with appreciate to different sorts of complexity measurements with embedded dimension $d = 3$ and time delay $l = 1$. *impe* additionally offers an alternate way of measuring similarity amongst patterns with appreciate to different sorts of entropy measurements, *impe* is calculated as in [16].

All the stated entropies have been calculated for 15360 pattern points, and have been divided into 6 home windows of 10 2d size (2560 samples), then they have been used to extract facets from the 19 EEG channels.

3 Statistical Analysis

The denoised 19 channels from the EEG dataset of the 15 HC, 15 S_MCI patients, and 5 VD sufferers have been preliminarily grouped into 5 recording areas that correspond to the scalp location of the cerebral cortex. These areas are the frontal vicinity the usage of (Fp1, Fp2, F3, F4, F7, F8, and Fz) channels, the temporal (T3 to T6) channels, the parietal (P3, P4, and Pz) channels, the occipital (O1 and O2) channels, and the central (C3, C4, and Cz) channels. Normality take a look at used to be then assessed the usage of the Kolmogorov–Smirnov test. Therefore, multivariate analyses of variance (MANOVA) used to be carried out as a statistical device by using the use of SPSS 25. MANOVA was used to determine whether the gender has affected in VD, S_MCI patients vs. HC over the brain regions. Four entropy-based features including *SpecEn*, *FuzEn*, *TsEn* and *impe* were set as dependent variables, whereas the gender (i.e. females and males), the group factor (i.e., HC, S_MCI, and VD) and the brain regions (i.e. frontal, temporal, parietal and occipital) were set as the independent variables.

4 Results and Discussion

The Savitzky-Golay (SG) filter was once adopted for smoothing and filtering the acquired EEG dataset. Figure 2 indicates the filtered sign and the authentic EEG sign on the equal graph, demonstrating that the effects of SG filter exhibit that the filtered sign has a smaller noise issue than the unique signal.

In this study, the gender differences for dementia patients have been investigated using *SpecEn*, *FuzEn*, *TsEn* and *impe* features. The two-way MANOVA has been conducted to report the interactions of gender and VD, S_MCI vs HC among the brain regions.

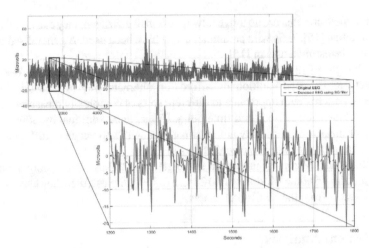

Fig. 2. F7 before and after using the SG as a denoising filter.

From Table 1 it can be observed that the HC and S_MCI and VD patients had a different pattern of brain complexity. In details, HC had higher entropy values in all brain regions compared to S_MCI and VD patients and that can be reported as ($SpecEn_{HC}$ > $SpecEn_{S\_MCI}$ > $SpecEn_{VD}$) using $SpecEn$, ($FuzEn_{HC}$ > $FuzEn_{S\_MCI}$ > $FuzEn_{VD}$) for $FuzEn$, ($TsEn_{HC}$ > $TsEn_{S\_MCI}$ > $TsEn_{VD}$) using $TsEn$ and ($impe_{HC}$ > $impe_{S\_MCI}$ > $impe_{VD}$) for $impe$. Interestingly, the HC females had higher complexity than the HC males in all brain regions whereas after getting cognitive impairment the complexity values for S_MCI and VD males in frontal, temporal, parietal, central and occipital brain regions are still complex and higher complexity values compare to S_MCI and VD females and that can mostly observed through $TsEn$ and $impe$ features.

Table 1. The impact of dementia varies by gender for the examined five scalp regions of the brain using $SpecEn$, $FuzEn$, $TsEn$ and $impe$.

Features	Subjects	Female					Male				
		Frontal	Temporal	Parietal	Central	Occipital	Frontal	Temporal	Parietal	Central	Occipital
SpecEn	HC	0.579	0.599	0.603	0.61	0.615	0.534	0.568	0.575	0.587	0.59
	S_MCI	0.566	0.592	0.596	0.608	0.593	0.527	0.55	0.563	0.577	0.574
	VD	0.527	0.547	0.551	0.576	0.548	0.525	0.545	0.547	0.566	0.542
FuzEn	HC	0.21	0.239	0.222	0.217	0.269	0.183	0.227	0.205	0.244	0.253
	S_MCI	0.175	0.195	0.18	0.199	0.217	0.177	0.209	0.194	0.203	0.232
	VD	0.172	0.192	0.172	0.174	0.204	0.176	0.19	0.184	0.186	0.205
TsEn	HC	3.555	3.538	3.574	3.556	3.55	3.492	3.499	3.522	3.508	3.481
	S_MCI	3.324	3.346	3.392	3.399	3.364	3.33	3.36	3.358	3.415	3.376
	VD	3.106	3.052	3.086	3.217	2.96	3.351	3.356	3.36	3.387	3.335
impe	HC	2.453	2.453	2.453	2.453	2.453	2.384	2.384	2.384	2.384	2.384
	S_MCI	2.354	2.354	2.354	2.354	2.354	2.36	2.36	2.36	2.36	2.36
	VD	2.131	2.131	2.131	2.131	2.131	2.333	2.333	2.333	2.333	2.333

5 Conclusion

In this study, gender differences of VD and S_MCI compared to HC over brain regions (i.e. frontal, temporal, parietal and occipital) were investigated. The SG filter was adopted for smoothing and filtering the acquired EEG dataset. The *SpecEn*, *FuzEn*, *TsEn* and *impe* were extracted from every EEG channel for different brain regions. MANOVA has been conducted to assess the gender differences over the brain regions for S_MCI and VD patients compared with HC subjects. Results show there were significant interactions of gender with dementia stages among the brain regions. Therefore, *SpecEn* reflected the slowing in the EEG signals of VD and S_MCI patients whereas *FuzEn*, *TsEn* and *impe* results in reducing the complexity in VD and S_MCI patients. As the EEG has been widely used as a potential tool in clinical practice due to its low cost and portability, it could become a reference that help to customize a specific therapeutic program to address the changes associated with S_MCI and VD. This study suggests that the entropy-based markers of EEG background activity in VD and S_MCI patients might be helpful in providing gender identifications indexes for VD detection. It can be concluded that the HC had higher entropy values in all brain regions compared to S_MCI and VD patients. Moreover, the HC females had higher complexity than the HC males in all brain regions whereas after getting cognitive impairment the complexity values for S_MCI and VD males in all brain regions become higher than the complexity values in females. This study had several limitations, like the sample size was small and in the future, an additional analysis with a large database should be performed.

References

1. Al-Qazzaz, N.K., et al.: Automatic artifact removal in EEG of normal and demented individuals using ICA–WT during working memory tasks. Sensors **17**(6), 1326 (2017)
2. Al-Qazzaz, N.K., et al.: Cognitive impairment and memory dysfunction after a stroke diagnosis: a post-stroke memory assessment. Neuropsychiatric disease and treatment **10**, 1677 (2014)
3. Al-Qazzaz, N.K., et al.: Role of EEG as biomarker in the early detection and classification of dementia. The Scientific World Journal, 2014. (2014)
4. Al-Qazzaz, N.K., Ali, S.H.M., Ahmad, S.A.: Differential Evolution Based Channel Selection Algorithm on EEG Signal for Early Detection of Vascular Dementia among Stroke Survivors. In: 2018 IEEE-EMBS Conference on Biomedical Engineering and Sciences (IECBES), IEEE. (2018)
5. Azami, H., et al.: Refined composite multiscale dispersion entropy and its application to biomedical signals. IEEE Trans. Biomed. Eng. **64**(12), 2872–2879 (2017)
6. Azami, H., Sanei, S.: Spike detection approaches for noisy neuronal data: assessment and comparison. Neurocomputing **133**, 491–506 (2014)
7. Azami, H., Rostaghi, M., Escudero, J.: Refined Composite Multiscale Dispersion Entropy: A Fast Measure of Complexity. arXiv preprint arXiv:1606.01379. (2016)
8. Escudero, J., et al.: Blind source separation to enhance spectral and non-linear features of magnetoencephalogram recordings. Application to Alzheimer's disease. Med. Eng. Phys. **31**(7), 872–879 (2009)

9. Al-Qazzaz, N.K., Ali, S.H.M., Islam, S., Ahmad, S.A., Escudero, J.: EEG wavelet spectral analysis during a working memory tasks in stroke-related mild cognitive impairment patients. In: Ibrahim, F., Usman, J., Mohktar, M.S., Ahmad, M.Y. (eds.) International Conference for Innovation in Biomedical Engineering and Life Sciences. IP, vol. 56, pp. 82–85. Springer, Singapore (2016). https://doi.org/10.1007/978-981-10-0266-3_17
10. Al-Qazzaz, N.K., et al.: Entropy-based markers of EEG background activity of stroke-related mild cognitive impairment and vascular dementia patients. In: 2nd International Conference on Sensors Engineering and Electronics Instrumental Advances (SEIA 2016), Barcelona, Spain. (2016)
11. Cirugeda-Roldan, E., et al.: Comparative study of entropy sensitivity to missing biosignal data. Entropy **16**(11), 5901–5918 (2014)
12. Simons, S., Espino, P., Abásolo, D.: Fuzzy entropy analysis of the electroencephalogram in patients with Alzheimer's disease: is the method superior to sample entropy? Entropy **20**(1), 21 (2018)
13. Havrda, J., Charvát, F.: Quantification method of classification processes. Concept Struct. *a*-entropy. Kybernetika **3**(1), 30–35 (1967)
14. Daróczy, Z.: Generalized information functions. Inf. Control **16**(1), 36–51 (1970)
15. Robert, S.: The Tsallis entropy of natural information. Phys. A: Stat. Mech. Appl. **386**(1), 101–118 (2007)
16. Morabito, F.C., et al.: Multivariate multi-scale permutation entropy for complexity analysis of Alzheimer's disease EEG. Entropy **14**(7), 1186–1202 (2012)

Endogenous Glucose Production Variation Assessment for Malaysian ICU Patients Based on Diabetic Status

A. A. Razak[1](✉), A. Abu-Samah[2], N. N. Razak[1], S. Baharudin[1], F. M. Suhaimi[3], and U. Jamaludin[4]

[1] College of Engineering, Universiti Tenaga Nasional, 43000 Kajang, Malaysia
athirahrazak@gmail.com
[2] Institute of Energy Infrastructure, Universiti Tenaga Nasional, 43000 Kajang, Malaysia
[3] Advanced Medical and Dental Institute, Universiti Sains Malaysia, Bertam, 13200 Kepala Batas, Penang, Malaysia
[4] Department of Mechanical Engineering, Universiti Malaysia Pahang, 26600 Pekan, Pahang, Malaysia

Abstract. Intensive Care Insulin-Nutrition-Glucose (ICING) model is used in Stochastic TARgeted (STAR) protocol to personalize glucose control in critically-ill patients. One of the important ICING parameters included in this physiological mathematical model is endogenous glucose production (EGP) which is defined as a constant value. EGP however may vary in individual patients and vary differently in critically-ill diabetic patients. This paper studies this aspect specifically to identify if certain EGP values will improve the estimation of insulin sensitivity (SI) through the reduction of unlikely SI estimation; SI = 0, blood glucose fit errors and simulated STAR glycaemic control performance. Analysis on 151 patients from two Malaysian hospitals, divided into 54 diabetic and 97 non-diabetic were done using 5 EGP values (1.16, 1.50, 2.00, 2.50, and 3.00) mmol/min to see the effect of EGP variations on both type of patients. The results indicate that the frequency of SI = 0 was improved with reduction, from 25.3% to 0.01% in diabetic and 13.4% to 0.008% in non-diabetic patients when EGP is raised from 1.16 mmol/min to 3.00 mmol/min. BG fit errors varied but with small variation and lower than 1%. The highest performance results of % blood glucose time in target range 6.0–10.0 mmol/L was obtained for EGP at 2.50 mmol/min, at 70.8% (diabetic) and EGP = 2.00 mmol/min, with 72.2% (non-diabetic). Overall results showed that choice of EGP values can have an impact on SI estimation and glycaemic control performance. Furthermore, certain EGP values have been identified to be beneficial to distinguish based on diabetic status.

Keywords: Diabetes · Glucose-insulin model · Endogenous glucose production · Glycaemic control · Insulin sensitivity

1 Introduction

Critically-ill diabetic and non-diabetic patients are commonly associated to stress hyperglycaemia [1]. These patients may have sepsis, hypertension, multiple organ failures and

© Springer Nature Switzerland AG 2021
F. Ibrahim et al. (Eds.): ICIBEL 2019, IFMBE Proceedings 81, pp. 129–136, 2021.
https://doi.org/10.1007/978-3-030-65092-6_15

worse higher rate of mortality [2, 3]. Hyperglycaemia occurs when insulin is no longer being produced or when it suppresses endogenous glucose production (EGP) due to high insulin resistance syndrome [4]. EGP plays an important role to sustain glycaemic level in diabetic and non-diabetic patients, where liver is the central production [5]. Over production of glucose by endogenous mechanism is the primary cause for type 2 diabetes [6].

ICING [7] is a clinically validated physiological model that enables insulin sensitivity (SI) estimation. The 'metabolic parameter' is identified hourly through integral fitting method [8] for a more personalized care as each individual in the ICU have different SI [9]. This model integrates EGP as one of its parameter and was built and validated based on New Zealand patients [7]. In a pilot trial for Malaysian Intensive Care Unit (ICU) patients [10], the patient's estimated SIs were generally lower than New Zealand's and Hungary's. Two unpublished studies showed that they also have larger sum of unlikely SI estimation, cases of SI = 0 or SI taking negative values. As the ICING model is designed using patients from a different demographic and with prevalence of diabetic status upon ICU admission, it is interesting to see if EGP estimation is one of the contributing factors to that difference in Malaysian critically-ill's SI estimation.

Stochastic TARgeted (STAR) [11, 12] protocol incorporates physiological ICING model [7, 13] as part of its glycaemic control. STAR is the latest transition control from conventional insulin therapy into an automated personalized care treatment [9]. The ICING model used in this control assumed a constant EGP value of 1.16 mmol/min based on steady state and unsuppressed by the insulin and glucose basal EGP [7].

Anane et al. [14] assessed several EGP values ranging between 1.5 to 3.5 mmol/min with step size 0.25 to improve ICING model SI estimation, through BG fitting errors quantification. The estimation method used by [14] suggested to be used only when there is negative SI values. Using 4 of the proposed EGP values with the lowest BG fit error and through quantification percentage of total number (nb.) for SI = 0 value, this study will assess if the variations of EGP will improve the SI = 0 estimation in both diabetic and non-diabetic critically-ill patients. Virtual simulations of Stochastic TARgeted (STAR) control were also performed to confirm if changes in SI will improve patient's performance and safety in Malaysian cohort.

2 Method

Retrospective data were separated into 54 diabetic (DM) and 97 non-diabetic (NDM) patients with similar distribution of age and length of stay, from Hospital Universiti Sains Malaysia (HUSM) and University Malaya Medical Centre (UMMC). Both hospitals used sliding scale glycaemic control. With 5 EGP values (1.16, 1.5, 2.0, 2.5, 3.0) data were used to run;

i)   BG fitting and estimation of SI
ii) STAR virtual simulation

Subjects demographic were categorized in Table 1 by total number of patients, age, total number of gender (%), length of ICU stays (days), and patient's diagnosis; hypertension (HPT), sepsis, kidney problems and others.

Table 1. Subjects Demographics.

Parameter	Median [IQR] when available		P-value similarity test
Type of patient	Diabetic	Non-diabetic	
Number of Patients	54 (35.8%)	97 (64.2%)	–
Age (years)	62 [57–66]	61 [50–69]	0.6632 > 0.05
% of Gender (F:M)	23 (42.5%): 31(57.5%)	34 (35%):63 (65%)	–
Length of Stay (days)	1.5 [3–6]	4 [2–7]	0.1088 > 0.05
Diagnosis			
- HPT	11	22	–
- Sepsis	14	18	–
- Kidney Problems	4	9	–
- Others	25	48	–

2.1 ICING Model

Intensive Care Insulin Nutrition Glucose (ICING) model is used to capture the highly dynamic metabolic parameter, SI. It is modeled using 7 equation as [7]. SI is identified hourly using integral fitting identification fitting method [15].

2.2 Insulin Sensitivity and BG Fitting Error Assessment

BG fit error is defined by the total percentage of absolute difference between measured and fitted BG. The equation for BG fit error is illustrated below,

$$\%BG_{fit,error} = \frac{|BG_{model} - BG_{measured}|}{BG_{measured}} \times 100\% \tag{8}$$

SI = 0 is physiologically irrelevant. SI is considered improved if the number of simulated SI = 0 using is reduced. ANOVA test was used to identify the significance of SI values distribution between the two EGP 1.16 mmol/min and 3.00 mmol/min of each cohort. P-value less than 0.05 is considered significant. Cumulative distribution frequency (CDF) of SI for both diabetic and non-diabetic cohorts was also executed to compare the pattern results.

2.3 Virtual Trial Analysis

STAR protocol [12] was used in a virtual trial to simulate glycemic control performance using ICING with modified EGPs. BG target range, insulin and nutrition administration were set based on Malaysian ICU protocol guidelines [16]. Targeted BG range was 6.0–10.0 mmol/L and range of insulin infusion was within 0.0–8.0 U/hr, with increment of 0.5 U–2.0 U. The nutrition input for patient's virtual trial was within 20–25 kcal/kg/day.

From virtual trial, median of BG and % time in BG target range (6.0–10.0 mmol/L) were assessed. Patient's safety metric was assessed by number of mild hypoglycaemia (BG < 4.4 mmol/L) and number of severe hypoglycaemia (BG < 2.2 mmol/L).

3 Results

3.1 Insulin Sensitivity and BG Fitting Error Assessment

Table 2 shows the percentage count of SI = 0 with 5 EGP values; 1.16, 1.50, 2.00, 2.50 and 3.00 mmol/min. Comparing EGP equal to 1.16 mmol/min and the highest proposed EGP of 3.00 mmol/min, the SI estimation improved significantly by reducing SI = 0 value from 25.3% to 0.01% (p-value < 0.05) for diabetic and 13.4% to 0.008% (p-value < 0.05) for non-diabetic patients. Status-wise comparison, diabetic patients have more SI = 0 compared to non-diabetic patients using all EGPs, but with 1.16 mmol/min the difference was the largest with 11.9%.

The table also shows the errors decreased from 0.79% to 0.40%, 0.47% to 0.62% and increase again to 0.79% when the elevated EGP values were set from 1.16 to 1.50, 2.00, 2.50 and 3.00 mmol/L respectively.

Table 2. Percentage of SI = 0 with EGP variations and the BG fit error results.

Patient's SI	Diabetic (Red)	Non-Diabetic (Blue)	Graphs
EGP 1.16 mmol/min	1468/5782=25.3%	1641/12177=13.4%	
EGP 1.50 mmol/min	316/5782=5.4%	371/12177=3.04%	
EGP 2.00 mmol/min	41/5782=0.7%	43/12177=0.3%	
EGP 2.50 mmol/min	5/5782=0.08%	13/12177=0.1%	
EGP 3.00 mmol/min	1/5782=0.01%	1/12177=0.008%	
ANOVA test	<0.05	<0.05	
BG Fit errors	**Diabetic**	**Non-Diabetic**	
EGP 1.16 mmol/min	0.79 [0.19-6.25]	0.62 [0.15 – 3.02]	
EGP 1.50 mmol/min	0.40 [0.36 -1.74]	0.37 [0.13- 1.12]	
EGP 2.00 mmol/min	0.47 [0.19-0.99]	0.48 [0.19 -1.13]	
EGP 2.50 mmol/min	0.62 [0.26-1.25]	0.64 [0.26-1.43]	
EGP 3.00 mmol/min	0.79 [0.32-1.56]	0.82 [0.32-1.75]	

Figures 1 shows the CDF of SI for (a) diabetic and (b) non-diabetic patients. The figures illustrate that SI with EGP = 1.16 mmol/min reaches the maximum faster than the rest of EGPs.

Figure 2 shows an example of a female diabetic patient's profile with 43 h of glycaemic control. The first and second panel show the clinical BG measurements, the model fitted BG and estimated SI according to different EGP values. Since this patient has diabetes, the initial BG reading of this patient was very high at 27.7 mmol/L, but it slowly decreased into stable zone within prescribed target range. The elevated EGP contributed in reducing the BG fit errors within the first 6 h, between 19–25 h and between 30–40 h. The SI = 0 are uniformly elevated with larger EGP values.

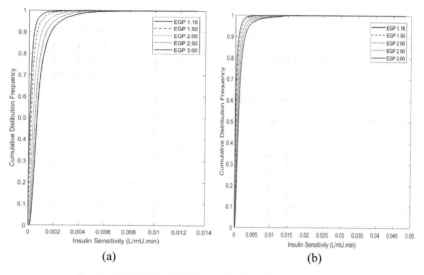

Fig. 1. SI CDF for (a) Diabetic (b) Non-diabetic patients.

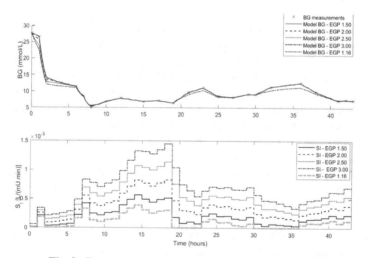

Fig. 2. Example of diabetic critically-ill patient's profiles.

3.2 Virtual Trial Analysis

Table 3 shows the performance in terms of median % BG time in band (TIB) 6.0–10.0 mmol/L range for diabetic and non-diabetic patients. The diabetic cohort median % BG in 6.0–10.0 mmol/L increased from 66.8% (EGP = 1.16) to 72.2% (EGP = 2.50) while, the non-diabetic cohort's increased from 70.7% (EGP = 1.16) to 72.8% (EGP = 2.00) and 72.2% (EGP = 2.50). The BG values reduced from 9.28 (EGP = 1.16) to 9.20 (EGP = 2.50) mmol/L and 7.95 (EGP = 1.16) to 7.81 (EGP = 2.50) mmol/L in diabetic and non-diabetic patients.

Patient safety for BG < 4.4 mmol/L shows number of cases reduced from 37 (EGP = 1.16) to 9 (EGP = 2.50) in diabetic and 38 (EGP = 1.16) to 20 (EGP = 3.00) in non-diabetic patients. Severe hypoglycaemic cases only occur on non-diabetic patients. The number were reduced from 6 (EGP = 1.16) to 3 and 4 using higher EGP values.

Table 3. Virtual trial performance and safety results.

EGP values	BG (mmol/L)		%BG TIB 6.0–10.0 mmol/L		Nb. of BG < 4.4 mmol/L		Nb. of BG < 2.2 mmol/L	
	DM	NDM	DM	NDM	DM	NDM	DM	NDM
EGP 1.16	9.28	7.95	66.8	70.7	37	38	0	6
EGP 1.50	9.30	7.86	66.1	71.8	10	30	0	4
EGP 2.00	9.23	7.82	65.2	72.8	14	25	0	4
EGP 2.50	9.20	7.81	70.8	72.2	9	23	0	3
EGP 3.00	9.20	7.81	63.7	71.7	12	20	0	4

4 Discussion

The variation of EGP as shown in Fig. 1 illustrates the linear increase of SI with each EGP values. Based on that, we can assume the estimation of SI for both diabetic and non-diabetic patients will continue to increase with higher EGP. However, higher EGP is not clinically relevant for ICU patients [17] thus EGP value is limited to 3.00 mmol/min in our study. In terms of the unlikely SI estimation, the number of SI = 0 reduced exponentially with increased values of EGP, and the maximum reduction is reached on EGP 3.00 mmol/min. The BG fit error has a 'V' trend. Minimum error was identified on EGP = 1.50 mmol/min, and the values keep rising onward. The differences between each EGP error is insignificant. Elevating EGP is beneficial to decrease SI = 0, but it needs to be compromised at least with BG fitting error. A further look at the STAR glycaemic control performance using this estimation showed that highest performance in target range is attributed to EGP = 2.50 mmol/min for diabetics but EGP = 2.00 mmol/min for non-diabetics. The number of cases for mild hypoglycaemia decreased with higher EGP value of 2.50 mmol/min and 3.00 mmol/min in diabetics and non-diabetics. While the variation of performance from non-diabetics is relatively the same. For EGP = 2.00 mmol/min and 2.50 mmol/min the performance is better in non-diabetic and diabetics. This question the existence of SI range that can improve Malaysian patient performance.

The SI non likely estimation recorded reduction from 25.3% (EGP = 1.16 mmol/min) to 0.01% (EGP = 3.00 mmol/min) and 13.4% (EGP = 1.16 mmol/min) to 0.008% (EGP = 3.00 mmol/min) in diabetic and non-diabetic patients. The difference is much more obvious in diabetics. Secondly, at EGP equals to 1.50 mmol/min, median BG fit errors between diabetics and non-diabetics recorded the largest gap from previous EGP value, 1.16 mmol/min with 0.39% and 0.25%. Again, the difference is more accentuated to the diabetics, but in both cases, the differences are larger at the beginning and start to slow down after. These results suggest to differentiate choice of EGP upon diabetic status only when working with the low 1.16 to 2.5 range. For cases with higher EGP, we can assume both cohorts can share the same constant for control and treatment recommendations. In any case, further studies need to be conducted to proof that the suggestion is solely based on diabetic status and not the available patient's data.

Based on this study, several orientations of improvement have been identified. First, simulation and discussion were done based on estimated SI using ICING model. The study was not supported by real SI that can be estimated using clinical techniques like homeostatic model assessment (HOMA) or glucose clamp technique. Second, based on the performance results, it is interesting to do a study on SI range that can improve Malaysian patient glycemic control performance. A feedback control within that range can give a better indication on the best choice of EGP. In any case, in depth study with more data needs to be done to validate any suggestion.

5 Conclusion

From this study, the EGP values between 1.50 and 2.50 mmol/min improved SI estimation and fitting error results in Malaysian diabetic and non-diabetic patients. Based on both cohorts' results, EGP values of 2.50 mmol/min strongly demonstrated the best compromised between reduction of SI = 0, BG fit error and % in target band of 6.0–10.0 mmol/L. The 1.50–2.50 mmol/min range of values can be proposed to be used as EGP constant in STAR Malaysia implementation to improve the automated treatment recommendation, thus ensuring a better performance and safety.

Acknowledgment. The research was enabled by UNITEN under BOLD grant. A special thanks to Dr Tan Ru Yi and Prof Dr. Mohd Shahnaz Hasan from University Malaya Medical Centre (UMMC), and Dr Mohd Zulfakar Mazlan from Hospital Universiti Sains Malaysia (HUSM) for the provision of data. Ethics were granted by National Institute of Health, Malaysia through UMMC and HUSM for this collaboration study with Universiti Sains Malaysia and Universiti Malaysia Pahang.

References

1. Ali Abdelhamid, Y., et al.: Stress hyperglycaemia in critically ill patients and the subsequent risk of diabetes: A systematic review and meta-analysis. Crit. Care **20**(1), 1–9 (2016)
2. Van den Berghe, G.: Beyond diabetes: saving lives with insulin in the ICU. Int. J. Obes. Relat. Metab. Disord. **26**(Suppl 3), S3–S8 (2002)
3. Dungan, K.M., Braithwaite, S.S., Preiser, J.C.: Stress hyperglycaemia. Lancet **373**(9677), 1798–1807 (2009)
4. Radziuk, J., et al.: Quantitation of basal endogenous glucose production in Type II diabetes: Importance of the volume of distribution, **45**(8) (2002)
5. Singhal, P., et al.: Regulation of endogenous glucose production after a mixed meal in type 2 diabetes. Am. J. Physiol. Metab. **283**(2), E275–E283 (2015)
6. DeFronzo, R.A.: Pathogenesis of type 2 diabetes mellitus. Med. Clin. North Am. **88**(4), 787–835 (2004)
7. Lin, J., et al.: A physiological Intensive Control Insulin-Nutrition-Glucose (ICING) model validated in critically ill patients. Comput. Methods Programs Biomed. **102**(2), 192–205 (2011)

8. Hann, C.E., et al.: Integral-based parameter identification for long-term dynamic verification of a Glucose-Insulin system model. Comput. Methods Programs Biomed. **77**(3), 259–270 (2005).
9. Chase, J.G., et al.: Next-generation, personalised, model-based critical care medicine: A state-of-the art review of in silico virtual patient models, methods, and cohorts, and how to validation them. Biomed. Eng. Online **17**(1), 24 (2018)
10. Abu-Samah, A., et al.: Model-based glycemic control in a Malaysian intensive care unit: performance and safety study. Med. Devices Evid. Res. **12**, 215–226 (2019)
11. Stewart, K.W., et al.: Nutrition delivery, workload and performance in a model-based ICU glycaemic control system. Comput. Methods Programs Biomed. **166**, 9–18 (2018)
12. Stewart, K.W., et al.: Safety, efficacy and clinical generalization of the STAR protocol: a retrospective analysis. Ann. Intensive Care **6**(1), 24 (2016)
13. Lin, J., et al.: Stochastic modelling of insulin sensitivity and adaptive glycemic control for critical care. Comput. Methods Programs Biomed. **89**(2), 141–152 (2008)
14. Anane, Y., et al.: Endogenous glucose production parameter estimation for intensive care patients. In: 2019 Scientific Meeting on Electrical-Electronics & Biomedical Engineering and Computer Science (EBBT), pp. 1–4 (2019)
15. Hann, C.E., et al.: Integral-based identification of patient specific parameters for a minimal cardiac model. Comput. Methods Programs Biomed. **81**(2), 181–192 (2006)
16. Malaysian Society of Intensive Care. Management Protocols In ICU Malaysia, September 2012
17. Pretty, C.: Analysis , classification and management of insulin sensitivity variability in a glucose-insulin system model for critical illness, thesis (2012)

Measurement of Prostate Gland: A Descriptive Study Among Asymptomatic Male Students in a Private University in Malaysia

M. L. Dinesh[1], N. M. Zain[1,2](✉) ⓘ, N. Balqis[1], and N. M. Mohammad[1]

[1] Medical Imaging Program, School of Health Sciences, KPJ Healthcare University College, 71800 Kota Seriemas, Negeri Sembilan, Malaysia
norhayati@kpjuc.edu.my

[2] Research Management Centre, KPJ Healthcare University College, 71800 Kota Seriemas, Negeri Sembilan, Malaysia

Abstract. Transabdominal ultrasound scan is one of the appropriate methods to measure the size of prostate gland. Enlarged prostate is a precursor to prostate cancer and hence, it is more of a concern when enlarged prostate occurs in young men. This study has been conducted to determine the actual size of prostate gland among asymptomatic male students in Malaysia and compare the volume of prostate gland among different age groups. A cross-sectional descriptive study was conducted among 101 male students aged between 18 to 26 years old in a private institution in Nilai, Negeri Sembilan, Malaysia. The respondents were randomly recruited using convenience sampling method. A validated self-administered questionnaire covering socio-demographic data was used. Respondents need to undergo a transabdominal ultrasound scanning by an expert in the measurement of prostate volume. Majority of the respondents were aged between 18 to 20 years old (55%) and were Malays (88%). A total of 92% of the respondents did not have any family history related to prostate cancer. The average size of prostate glands was found to be normal in size with 21.1 ($\pm$3.9) cc. Prostate dimension for students aged 18–20 years old was significantly smaller compared to respondent aged 24–26 years old (p = 0.01). It is concluded that, the asymptomatic male students in this study has normal size of prostate gland.

Keywords: Prostate gland · Prostatic volume · Ultrasound scanning

1 Introduction

The prostate gland is a conical fibromuscular, single accessory structure of the male reproductive system. It envelops the urethra in the pelvic cavity. The prostate is situated just above the pelvic floor, inferior to the urinary bladder, posterior to the pubic symphysis, and anterior to the rectum. The prostate comprises as 30–40 individual complex glands, which develop from the urethral epithelium into the neighboring wall of the urethra [1]. The transverse measurement of prostatic base is about 4 cm. The gland measures around 2 cm antero-posteriorly and 3 cm in its vertical diameters. The estimated

© Springer Nature Switzerland AG 2021
F. Ibrahim et al. (Eds.): ICIBEL 2019, IFMBE Proceedings 81, pp. 137–141, 2021.
https://doi.org/10.1007/978-3-030-65092-6_16

weight of prostate gland is about 8 g in younger adults, but almost constantly enlarges with the progression of benign prostatic hyperplasia (BPH): it generally weighs 40 g, but occasionally as high as 150 g or even higher, after the first five decades of life [2].

The zonal anatomy of the prostate is clinically significant because most carcinomas occur in the peripheral zone, whereas BPH affects the transitional zone, which may develop to make the bulk of the prostate. BPH begins as micronodules in the transitional zone which grow and consolidate to form macro-nodules around the inferior margin of the pre-prostatic urethra, just above the verumontanum. The central zone encircling the ejaculatory ducts is hardly affected by any illness [1].

In men between the age of 21 and 30 years, the normal prostate reaches 20 ± 6 g, and its weight remains virtually consistent with increasing age unless BPH develops. The prevalence of pathological BPH is only 8% at the fourth decade; however, 50% of the male population has pathological BPH when they are 51 to 60 years old [3].

The size of prostate gland can be measured through the transabdominal approach with excellent images and reasonable accuracy, as it is atraumatic and well tolerated by the patient. It does not require special additional equipment, hence making it a procedure that can be performed in all ultrasound laboratories. It is considered to be fast and easy, and the prostate is visualized in two planes providing the three dimensions necessary for accurate measurement [4, 5].

Literatures has reported the dimension of normal prostate gland; nonetheless, limited studies done had focused on measuring normal prostate gland in asymptomatic young males. Hence, this study has been conducted to determine the actual size of prostate gland among asymptomatic male students in Malaysia. Besides, it is to compare size of prostate gland among asymptomatic male students between age groups.

2 Methodology

This cross sectional study conducted at a private University, Malaysia for one year from July 2017 to July 2018. This study was approved by Institutional Review Board with ethical registered number (KPJUC/RMC/BPH/EC/2017/122). A total of 101 asymptomatic male students recruited aged between 18 to 26 years old. The students with history of prostate surgery or congenital anomalies of prostate gland were excluded from the study.

2.1 Data Collection Tools

Two type of data collection sheets; (1) a self-administered form of questions on socio-demographic characteristics such as age, race and family history of prostatic diseases, and (2) prostate gland dimension measurement form for transabdominal ultrasonography procedure which includes the anteroposterior (length), cephalocaudal (height) and transverse (width) measurements of prostate gland were used. Prostatic transabdominal ultrasound was done using ultrasound machine (Esoate, MyLabTMOne Model) with a convex abdominal transducer (5–13 MHz). The ultrasound scan was performed by an expert with a minimum of five years experience in the field of medical ultrasonography.

2.2 Data Collection Process

The respondents were briefed about the whole procedure and they were consented prior to it. The socio-demographic form should be answered by each respondent before they underwent transabdominal ultrasound scan. Respondent was asked to drink at least 500 ml of water and wait until the urinary bladder was adequately filled; approximately about 30 min. The full bladder serves as an acoustic window to better visualize the prostate gland. Three measurements of prostate gland were done and recorded in the measurement form, which includes anteroposterior (length), cephalocaudal (height) and transverse (width) measurements of prostate. The mean of each measurement was used for further analysis. The ultrasound scan images were stored in the archive for further reference.

2.3 Statistical Analysis

The data collected were analyzed using the statistical package for social science (SPSS) version 22.0 and Microsoft Excel version 16.0 (Microsoft Office 365). The prostate gland volume was calculated by using the ellipsoid formula (1), and One Way *ANOVA* test was used to compare the prostate volume between age groups.

$$\text{Prostate Volume} = W \times H \times L \times \frac{\pi}{6} \tag{1}$$

W = Width *(Transverse measurement)*
H = Height *(Cephalocaudal measurement)*
L = Length *(Anteroposterior measurement)*

3 Results

Total of 101 questionnaire was fully completed. Table 1 shows the demographic data contains the age, race and family history of prostate diseases of respondents. Table 2 shows the mean prostatic dimensions of respondents.

Table 1. Socio-Demographic Characteristics of Respondent.

Demographic data	Criteria	N (%)
Age group	18–20 years old	56 (55.5)
	21–23 years old	28 (27.7)
	24–26 years old	17 (16.8)
Race	Malay	89 (88.1)
	Chinese	2 (2.0)
	Indian	6 (5.9)
	Others	4 (4.0)
Family History	Yes	8 (7.9)
	No	93 (92.1)

Table 2. Mean Measurements of the Prostate Dimensions and Volume.

Age Group (years)	Height (cm) Mean (SD)	Width (cm) Mean (SD)	Length (cm) Mean (SD)	Prostate Volume (cc) Mean (SD)	Total Volume of Prostate (cc) Mean (SD)
18–20	2.64 (0.27)	3.66 (0.38)	4.02 (0.41)	20.42 (3.14)	21.07 (3.86)
21–23	2.65 (0.28)	3.68 (0.31)	4.07 (0.43)	20.88 (4.29)	
24–26	2.74 (0.34)	3.86 (0.34)	4.21 (0.43)	23.52 (4.49)	

One-way ANOVA was done to compare the mean of prostate volume among the three age groups. The respondents of 24 to 26 years age group have the greatest volume of prostate gland (mean: 23.52; SD: 4.49) and the respondents of 18 to 20 years age group have the least volume of prostate gland (mean: 20.41; SD: 3.14). The post-hoc tests shows that prostate volume between age group 18 to 20 and 24 to 26 years old was significantly different ($p < 0.01$). The result proves that the prostate volume would increase with age and prostate dimension for respondents aged 18–20 years old was significantly smaller compared to respondents aged 24–26 years old ($p < 0.01$).

4   Discussion

According to Edwards (2008), the normal size of the prostate gland was 20 to 30 cc [6]. The prevalence of symptomatic benign prostate enlargement (BPE) in Malaysia was 39.3%. This prevalence increased 8% per decade from 41.7% for men aged 50 to 59 to 65.4% for men aged 70 or more [7]. The Star Malaysia (2017), reported that in Malaysia, BPE only occurs after the age of 40, where the exact cause has not been identified, but it is believed to be due to the imbalance of sex hormones. Strong evidence that decreasing levels of androgens, as happens in older age, alters genes which control apoptosis, which is programmed cell death. This leads to an overgrowth of cells in the prostate [8]. In our study, the entire population was less than 30 years old and the study reveals that the average size of the prostate gland is 21 cc, which is well placed below the normal limit of this age groups.

The prostate dimension of students aged 18–20 years old was significantly smaller compared to respondents aged 24–26 years old. This is supported by Gray's anatomy (2014), which explained that the prostate gland begins a developmental stage between the ages of roughly 14 and 18 years and enlarges more than doubles in volume. The follicular development is the main reason for the growth, partially from terminal-buds on ducts, and slightly from alteration of the ductal branches [2].

During the third decade the glandular epithelium grows by irregular multiplication of the epithelial infoldings into the lumen of the follicles. After the third decade, the size of the prostate remains nearly unchanged until 45–50 years. After 45–50 years the prostate tends to develop BPH: an age-related condition. If when a man lives long enough then BPH is inevitable but it is not always symptomatic.

The significant increase of human prostatic growth with age has been reported by many journals. Our study also found that there was a significant increase in the volume of prostate gland with the age. Moreover, a study conducted by Hoo et al. (2012), also reported that the normal volume of prostate gland range about 0.25 cc at birth to 10 cc sized at puberty [9]. After puberty, the prostate volume will continuously grow as the age increase for most of the male's life. Findings from Zhang et al. (2013), shows that the increase in prostate volume was measurable in each 10-year age group and doubled from 5.5 ml in 40–49 years to 11.1 ml in 70–80 years [10]. Furthermore, males aged between 50 and 57 had the highest volume of the prostate gland (28.89 cc), while the lowest prostatic volume was among the age 30 years old and below (19.97 cc) [11].

5 Conclusion

It is concluded that the asymptomatic male students in this study has normal size of prostate gland. Students aged 18–20 years old has smaller prostate dimension compared to students aged 24–26 years old.

Acknowledgement. This research work is supported by the KPJ Healthcare University College [Grant number: KPJUC/RMC/BPH/EC/2017/122]. Authors would also like to express their heartfelt gratitude to the respondents who participated in the study.

References

1. Standring, S.: Gray's Anatomy. The Anatomical Basis of Clinical Practice, 40th ed. Churchill Livingstone (2008)
2. Drake, R.L., Vogl, A.W., Mitchell, A.W.: Gray's Anatomy for Students, Third Edition. Gray's Anatomy for Students (2015)
3. Berry, S.J., Coffey, D.S., Walsh, P.C., Ewing, L.L.: The Development of Human Benign Prostatic Hyperplasia with Age. J. Urol. **132**, 474–479 (1984)
4. Henneberry, M., Carter, M.F., Neiman, H.L.: Estimation of Prostatic Size by Suprapubic Ultrasonography. J. Urol. **121**, 615–616 (1979)
5. Abu-Yousef, M.M., Narayana, A.S.: Transabdominal ultrasound in the evaluation of prostate size. J. Clin. Ultrasound **10**, 275–278 (1982)
6. Edwards, J.L.: Diagnosis and management of benign prostatic hyperplasia. Am. Fam. Phys. **77**, 1403 (2008)
7. Teh, G.C., et al.: Prevalence of symptomatic BPE among Malaysian men aged 50 and above attending screening during prostate health awareness campaign. Med. J. Malaysia **56**, 186–195 (2001)
8. The prostate can leave you prostrate. The Star Malaysia, pp. 1–5 (2017)
9. Hoo, N.K., Ayob, M.A., Salim, M.I.M., Pahl, C., Abduljabbar, H.N., Supriyanto, E.: Prostate volume Ultrasonography: the Relationship of body weight, height, body mass index and ethnicity in transabdominal measurement. Int. J. Biol. Biomed. Eng. **6**(4), 187–95 (2012)
10. Zhang, S.-J., et al.: Relationship between age and prostate size. Asian J. Androl. **15**, 116–120 (2013)
11. Ebeye, A., Oyem, J., Iweariulor, B., Ubah, S.: Ultrasonographic assessment of normal prostate volume and splenic length among Urhobo ethnic group in Delta State of Nigeria. Ann. Bioanthropology **4**(2), 101 (2017)

Common Mammographic Positioning Error in Digital Era

Norhashimah Mohd Norsuddin$^{(\boxtimes)}$ ⓘ and Zhi Xuan Ko

Diagnostic Imaging and Radiotherapy Programme, Faculty of Health Sciences, Universiti Kebangsaan Malaysia (UKM), Kuala Lumpur Campus, 50300 Kuala Lumpur, Malaysia
norhashimahnorsuddin@ukm.edu.my, zhixuan0517@hotmail.my

Abstract. Although digital technology increases cancer detection rate, the quality of mammographic images still relies on how the breast is being positioned during the procedure. This study determined the association between type of positioning errors and false negative mammogram found in digital mammography. **Methods:** Image quality of 17 false negative (FN) digital mammographic cases was independently evaluated by one radiologist using the PGMI criteria. The type of positioning errors made in each mammogram was identified. Chi-square test was used to analyse the association between the type of positioning errors made and FN mammogram. **Results:** Image quality was significantly different for all mammographic views in digital mammograms, $\chi^2 = 29.168$, p < 0.0001. Majority of mammograms had moderate quality image (41.9%), followed by G grade (25.8%), I grade (17.7%) and P grade (14.5%). A significant association was seen between the positioning error with insufficient pectoral muscles projected and mammographic views, $\chi^2 = 17.956$, $p < 0.05$. However, no significant association was demonstrated for other positioning errors ($p > 0.05$). Errors such as not well demonstrated inframammary fold was the most common positioning errors found in mediolateral oblique view. Contrarily, insufficient projection of pectoral muscles alone was the most common positioning error made in craniocaudal view with 94.1% and 92.9% for left and right side respectively. **Conclusion:** Image quality of false negative mammogram is appreciably impacted by breast positioning error. Improper positioning could lead to inaccurate and less precision interpretation by radiologists. Thus, improper positioning affecting most of missed breast cancer in screening mammography. A high mammographic technique is crucial for cancer to be early and successfully detected.

Keywords: Mammography · PGMI · Positioning error · False negative

1 Introduction

Early detection of breast cancer has been proven to make a significant difference in quality of life, disease progression and mortality rates [1, 2]. With availability of digital technology in medical imaging, an increment in cancer detection rate has been proven when using digital mammography particularly in breast with high mammographic density [3, 4]. The use of post processing tools may allow greater capability to differentiate

© Springer Nature Switzerland AG 2021
F. Ibrahim et al. (Eds.): ICIBEL 2019, IFMBE Proceedings 81, pp. 142–149, 2021.
https://doi.org/10.1007/978-3-030-65092-6_17

normal tissue from cancer by highlighting suspicious regions of interest from dense fibroglandular background [5, 6]. It is possible, therefore, that with digital technology the concern over lesions being obscured with dense fibroglandular tissue may no longer be justified.

Despite the advances of digital technology in mammography, a high-quality mammography is still imperative for a reliable detection and accurate characterization of subtle lesions in the breast [7]. The quality of the mammographic images depends critically on the positioning of the breast, compression, optimum exposure, sharpness, noise, and contrast [8]. The positioning technique in mammography poses a few challenges due to the varying age, sizes, and body habitus of the patient [9]. In fact, positioning the breast during mammography procedure merely operator dependent.

Previous study has demonstrated that malpositioned breast contributed the largest portion of missed cancer in technical aspects [1]. Hence, breast positioning plays an essential role in maintaining the quality of mammogram and reducing the false negative mammography diagnosis particularly in this digital era. However, very limited studies have been carried out to evaluate the association between the positioning errors and false negative mammography particularly in this digital era. Therefore, identifying the quality images and common type of positioning errors of missed cancer warrant further investigations. In this study, the association between the type of positioning errors and false negative diagnosis was also investigated.

2 Materials and Methods

Ethics approval was granted by Institutional Research Board (NN-2018-080). Mammography reports of the patients were reviewed in the Radiology Information System (RIS) and the mammograms were retrieved through OsiriX DICOM viewer system.

2.1 Case Selection

A total of 17 false negative (FN) mammographic cases were retrospectively identified from the clinical database for this study. Each FN case was then grouped according to four standards mammographic views; including left craniocaudal (LCC), left mediolateral oblique (LMO), right craniocaudal (RCC), right mediolateral oblique (RMLO). All mammographic cases were taken using full-field detector digital mammography Lorad Selenia by Hologic. A false negative (FN) case is defined when cancer is detected in the mammogram which was initially a negative or benign mammography (Breast Imaging Reporting and Data System (BIRADS) 1–2) within two-year follow-up mammography. Cases with unilateral and bilateral mammographic views (CC and MLO) and histopathologically-proven positive cases were included in this study. Patient with breast implant, absence of CC or MLO views in any side of breast without mastectomy or no histopathological results were also excluded from this study. All BIRADS category for each FN cases were also identified.

2.2 PGMI Classification

The image quality of FN case was independently evaluated using PGMI system by one consultant radiologist with more than 10 years' experience in reporting radiography. Each positive case was classified as perfect (P grade), good (G grade), moderate (M grade) or inadequate (I grade) respectively. The presence of specific positioning errors in mammogram was also identified for each case. Other mammography image quality criteria such as compression, exposure, sharpness, correct image processing and artefacts were not evaluated in this study.

2.3 Statistical Analysis

The proportion of image quality (P, G, M, I) between different mammographic views were analysed. The association between type of positioning errors and the false negative mammogram was computed using Chi-square test. In addition, the proportion of BIRADS category between different PGMI image quality was also computed using Chi-square test. All the statistical analyses were done using Statistical Package for the Social Sciences (SPSS, version 25) and statistical significance was determined at a p-value < 0.05.

3 Results

From 17 FN cases, 17 mammograms of left breast and 14 mammograms of right breast were available for review and were categorized into four PGMI image quality classifications (Table 1). Analysis using Fisher's Exact Test showed that the proportion of FN cases graded for image quality is significantly different for all mammographic views, $\chi^2 = 29.168$, p < 0.0001. Majority of FN mammograms had moderate image quality (41.9%), followed by G (25.8%), I (17.7%) and P (14.5%). For left breast, LCC and LMLO mammograms were mostly graded in M with 47.1% and 58.8% respectively. This was followed by G (47.1%) and I grade (11.8%) for LCC and, P (23.5%) and I grade (17.6%) for LMLO. None of the mammograms were identified with any positioning error in LCC or G grade in LMLO. For the right breast, most of the FN cases had image quality of G (64.3%), followed by M (14.3%), I (14.3%) and P grade (7.1%) in RCC view. For RMLO view, 42.9% of the mammograms had M grade and 28.6% for each I and P grade but no mammogram with G grade was identified.

Insufficient projection of the pectoral muscles was the most common positioning error in CC view for both left (94.1%) and right (92.9%) sides. Insufficient inclusion of breast tissues on the image followed as the second most attribute positioning error found in the CC view with 11.8% in LCC and 14.3% in RCC. The least common positioning error made in CC view was nipple not in profile and it was only found in left breast (5.9%). For MLO view, inframammary fold not well demonstrated was the most likely type of positioning error seen in both LMLO (70.6%) and RMLO (64.3%). This was followed by insufficient projection of pectoral muscles (52.9%) and insufficient projection of breast tissues (17.6%) in LMLO. However, the percentage of positioning error with insufficient projection of breast tissues was higher than insufficient projection

Table 1. Proportion of false negative mammograms graded for PGMI image quality between different mammographic views.

Mammographic view of FN	PGMI image quality, n (%)				Total, n (%)	χ^2	P value
	P	G	M	I			
LCC	0 (0.0)	7 (41.2)	8 (47.1)	2 (11.8)	17 (100)		
LMLO	4 (23.5)	0 (0.0)	10 (58.8)	3 (17.6)	17 (100)		
RCC	1 (7.1)	9 (64.3)	2 (14.3)	2 (14.3)	14 (100)	29.168	< 0.001*
RMLO	4 (28.6)	0 (0.0)	6 (42.9)	4 (28.6)	14 (100)		
Total	9 (14.5%)	16 (25.8)	26 (41.9)	11 (17.7)	62 (100)		

¥FN = False negative, LCC = Left craniocaudal, LMLO = Left mediolateral oblique, RCC = Right craniocaudal, RMLO = Right mediolateral oblique
*statistically significant difference at $p < 0.05$, *Fisher's Exact Test*

Table 2. Association of positioning errors and false negative mammograms in both craniocaudal and mediolateral oblique views of right and left breast.

Type of positioning error	Mammographic view of FN cases, n (%)				Total mammographic images, n (%)	χ^2	P value
	LCC	LMLO	RCC	RMLO			
Pectoral muscles insufficiently projected, n (%)							
Insufficient	16 (94.1)	9 (52.9)	13 (92.9)	5 (35.7)	43 (69.4)	17.956	<0.05*
Sufficient	1 (5.9)	8 (47.1)	1 (7.1)	9 (64.3)	19 (30.6)		
Nipple in profile							
No	1 (5.9)	0 (0.0)	0 (0.0)	1 (7.1)	2 (3.2)	2.214	0.847
Yes	16 (94.1)	17 (100.0)	17 (100.0)	13 (92.9)	60 (96.8)		
Insufficient breast tissue projected, n (%)							
Insufficient	2 (11.8)	3 (17.6)	2 (14.3)	6 (42.9)	13 (21.0)	4.652	0.214
Sufficient	15 (88.2)	14 (82.4)	12 (85.7)	8 (57.1)	49 (79.0)		
Inframammary fold not well demonstrated, n (%)							
No	–	12 (70.6)	–	9 (64.3)	21 (67.7)		0.999
Yes	–	5 (29.4)	–	5 (29.4)	10 (32.3)		

*statistically significant difference at $p < 0.05$, Fisher's Exact Test

of pectoral muscles in RMLO (42.9% vs 35.7%). Improper positioning of nipple was the least common error made in MLO view with 7.1% found in right side only. Analysis of Fisher's exact test (Table 2) indicated a significant association between the type of positioning error with insufficient pectoral muscles projected and mammographic views, $\chi^2 = 17.956, p < 0.05$. However, no significant association was demonstrated for other positioning errors ($p > 0.05$). BIRADS category was not associated with the different types of PGMI image quality $\chi^2 = 13.561, p = 0.197$, Fisher's Exact Test (Table 3). M grade mammograms consisted of 100.0% BIRADS 3, 43.3% BIRADS 4, 38.9% BIRADS 4c and 50% BIRADS 5. While 15% I grade was more likely to have higher BIRADS category (4–5). All FN mammograms did not have positioning error type of presence of skinfold in the image.

Table 3. Association of BIRADS category between different PGMI image quality.

PGMI image quality classification	BIRADS category, n (%)					Total, n (%)	χ^2	P value
	3	4a	4c	4	5			
Perfect	0 (0.0)	2 (50.0)	3 (16.3)	4 (13.3)	0 (0.0)	9 (15.0)	13.561	0.197
Good	0 (0.0)	2 (50.0)	7 (38.9)	6 (20.0)	1 (25.0)	16 (26.7)		
Moderate	4 (100.0)	0 (0.0)	7 (38.9)	13 (43.3)	2 (50.0)	26 (43.3)		
Inadequate	0 (0.0)	0 (0.0)	1 (5.6)	7 (23.3)	1 (25.0)	9 (15.0)		

BIRADS = Breast Imaging-Reporting and Data System

4   Discussion

A significant association between the image quality and mammographic views demonstrated in this study explains that poor image quality of mammogram can be linked to undetected breast cancer. Overall clinical image quality of missed cancer cases in this study has poor positioning technique with more than 50% were graded as M and I grade. The image quality of mammogram also failed to achieve the acceptable quality standard in accordance to the quality assurance of Ministry of Health in Malaysia [10], whereby mammograms with P, G, M grades only constituted to 90% in this study (< 97% requirement). It is recommended that P and G grade should constitute to more than 50% and images with I grade should be less than 3%, however, our results showed undesirable results with 35% and 8% respectively.

Although M grade mammogram is often considered acceptable for diagnostic purposes, it is still known as poor positioned mammogram with one or more errors. Due to these positioning errors, some portion of breast tissue may not be completely imaged on the mammogram and evaluated by the radiologist or breast reader. Thus, cancer in that particular portion of the breast is more likely to be missed. The sensitivity of mammography will therefore decrease significantly. Indeed, the sensitivity of mammography dropped from 84.4% among cases with good positioning to 66.3% among cases with poor positioning [11], Furthermore, poor image quality have been found responsible for delayed detection in 22% of screening-detected cancers and 35% of interval breast cancers [12], Delayed cancer detection will result in diagnosis of cancer at a more advanced stage and reduce chances of survival among patients. We found that all the missed breast cancer in this study had a high BIRADS category (3, 4, 4a, 4c and 5) with more than 55% attributed to poor image quality (M and I grade). The chance of being diagnosed with breast cancer increases with the rise in BIRADS category. With some of characteristics of mammographic lesion features being challenging to detect [13], a poor clinical image quality therefore will increase the likelihood of the breast cancer being missed and delay the early treatment delivered. As for a very poorly positioned mammogram (I grade), a repeat mammography is required, resulting in increased radiation exposure to the patient.

An ideal CC view should demonstrate maximum amount of medial and lateral breast tissue with retromammary space and some portion of pectoral muscle. Posterior medial breast tissues and pectoral muscles are important to be included in CC view given that undetected cancers are more frequently located at these regions in women at high risk [14]. Unfortunately, insufficient projection of pectoral muscles and inclusion of posterior breast tissues are the most common positioning error found in CC as compared to MLO view in this study. Positioning of the pectoral muscle during mammography were deemed the most challenging part in mammography technique with a significant association demonstrated in this study ($P < 0.05$). Importantly, the pectoral muscles were only visualised on 30%–40% of cases in CC view when the breast was properly positioned [15]. Visualisation of pectoral muscles on CC view will assure the inclusion of posterior part of breast tissue.

A high quality MLO mammogram should have sufficient visualisation of pectoral muscles, well demonstrated IMF, nipple in profile and no skin fold or artefacts seen [16, 17]. This mammographic view best visualizes the posterior and upper-quadrants of the breast. However, among all missed cancer cases from MLO view in this study, majority were graded as M grade and reflected a number of positioning errors including not well demonstrated IMF, insufficient projection of pectoral muscles and breast tissues. A previous study also found that 5.6% of the missed cancer was caused by the poor positioning of mammography especially if pectoral muscles and IMF were insufficiently projected [18]. Inability to visualize these particular breast area may increase the likelihood of missing an invasive breast cancer and reduce the sensitivity of mammography [18, 19]. Although, the true incidence of breast cancer found in the IMA is not well known [20], the presence of IMF is still a very important indication that the postero-inferior part of breast tissues has been sufficiently imaged. Anatomical presentation and the ability of the radiographer to manoeuvre the breast prior and during the mammography procedure is known to attribute to the extent the IMF is included on the image [21], ultimately influencing the final grade awarded.

Failure in demonstrating the IMF in MLO view showed a significant association with missed cancer in the current study. Previous studies have stated that there is a constant relationship between the IMF and the inferior origin of the pectoralis major muscles that coincides with the embryologic development of the chest wall [22, 23]. Hence, when the chest wall muscles contract and not in a relaxed state; IMF and the pectoralis major muscles are linked and will be attracted towards the chest wall, making the breast positioning ever more difficult. Often, when positioning for MLO projection, the radiographers are not only positioning the breast but also required to adjust the patient's body and the placement of image receptor to ensure whole MLO image criteria can be visualised.

Regardless how advance the technology is, a good clinical skill still plays an imperative role in maximizing the number of breast cancer being detected in mammography. A skilful radiographer can minimize the errors made and likelihood of cancer being missed. The importance of training, via continued education should be emphasized among the radiographers and technologists. Furthermore, a systematic assessment of image quality in screening mammography program at the centres should be employed in daily practice.

It is acknowledged that an important limitation of this study is that the image quality evaluation using PGMI classifications system was done by one radiologist which may introduce bias in the study. In addition, the PGMI classification system has a subjective factor despite recommendations, criteria and guidelines. This limitation can be overcome in the future study by having the scoring system for each PGMI criteria and increase the subcategories of the criteria with more than one evaluator. Future research which involves a bigger sample size and reduce the significant effect of common mistakes made in a specific centre on the statistical analysis.

5 Conclusion

Overall clinical image quality of missed cancer cases in this study has poor positioning technique with more than 50% were graded as M and I grade. A significant association was demonstrated between the image quality and mammographic views. The common positioning errors found in CC view was insufficient visualization of posteromedial tissue and incorrect IMA not well demonstrated contributed to the most attribute positioning error in MLO view. Hence, the findings suggested that mammographic procedures are highly operator dependent to produce high diagnostic quality images. Poor clinical image quality could affect the image interpretation and delay the diagnosis of breast cancer. Thus, the effectiveness of breast cancer screening program fails to meet it purpose. A dedicated training can be tailored for radiographers that likely to make those positioning errors. Through this training, the radiographers' performance may improve as well as the mammography quality services.

References

1. Rasha, M.K., Naglaa, M.A.R., Hassan, M.A.: Missed Breast Carcinoma; Why and How to Avoid? J. Egyptian Nat. Cancer Inst. 19(3), 178–194 (2007)

2. Aidalina, M., Syed, M.A.: The uptake of Mammogram screening in Malaysia and its associated factors: a systematic review. Med. J. Malaysia 73(4), 202–211 (2018)
3. Heddson, B., et al.: Digital versus screen-film mammography: a retrospective comparison in a population-based screening program. Eur. J. Radiol. 64(3), 419–425 (2007)
4. Chelliah, K.K., Voon, N.S.M.F., Ahamad, H.: Breast density: does it vary among the main ethnic groups in Malaysia? Open J. Med. Imaging 3(4), 105–109 (2013)
5. Kanaga, K.C., Yap, H.H., Laila, S.E., Sulaiman, T., Zaharah, M., Shantini, A.A.: A critical comparison of three full field digital mammography systems using figure of merit. Med. J. Malaysia 65(2), 119–122 (2010)
6. Chelliah, K.K., Wee, C.A., Elias, L.S., Aziz, S.: Image quality of two full field digital mammography using a female breast phantom. J. Sains Kesihatan Malaysia (Malaysian Journal of Health Sciences) 7(1), 65–72 (2009)
7. Yaffe, M.J. et al.: Technical aspects of image quality in Mammography. J. ICRU 9(2), 33–51 (No 2 Report 82)
8. Manju, B.P., et al.: Breast Positioning during Mammography: Mistakes to be Avoided. Breast Cancer Basic Clin. Res. 8, 119–124 (2014)
9. Olive, P., Positioning chanllenges in Mammography. Radiol. Tech. 85(4), 417–439M (2014)
10. Malaysia, Quality Assurance Guidelines in Radiology Service. Act 304, 2017
11. Taplin, S.H., et al.: Screening mammography: clinical image quality and the risk of interval breast cancer. Am. J. Roentgenol. 178, 797–803 (2002)
12. Ashley, I.H., Kelly, L.O., Jason, B.G.: Mammography positioning standards in the digital era: is the status quo acceptable? Am. J. Roentgenol. 209, 1–7 (2017)
13. Norsuddin, N.M., et al.: An investigation into the mammographic appearances of missed breast cancers when recall rates are reduced. British J. Radiol. 90(1076), 20170048 (2017)
14. Min, S.B., Woo, K.M., Jung, M.C.: Breast cancer detected with screening US: reasons for nondetection at Mammography. Radiology 270(2), 369–377 (2014)
15. Robyn, L.: Digital Mammography: clinical image evaluation. Breast Imaging, An Issue of Radiologic Clinics of North America (2010)
16. England, P.H.: NHS Breast Screening Programme Guidance for breast screening Mammographers (2017) Third edition
17. Peitgen, H.O.: Digital Mammography: IWDM 2002 6th International Workshop on Digital Mammography, Springer, Berlin (2002)
18. Muttarak, M., Pojchamarnwiputh, S., Chaiwun, B.: Breast carcinomas: why are they missed? Singapore Med. J. 47, 851–857 (2006)
19. Kamal, R.M., et al.: Missed breast carcinoma; why and how to avoid? J. Egypt Natl. Cancer Inst. 19, 178–194 (2007)
20. Behranwala, K.A., Gui, P.H.: Breast cancer in the inframammary fold: is preserving the inframammary fold during mastectomy justified. Breast J. 11, 340–342 (2002)
21. Bassett, L.W., et al.: Mammographic positioning: evaluation from the view box. Breast Imaging 188(3), 803–806 (1993)
22. Netscher, D.T., Peterson, R.: Normal and abnormal development of the extremities and trunk. Clin. Plast. Surg. 17(1), 13–21 (1990)
23. Nanigian, B.R., Granger, B.: Inframammary crease: positional relationship to the pectoralis major muscle origin. Aesthetic Surgery J. 27(5), 509–512 (2007)

A Dot-Probe Paradigm for Attention Bias Detection in Young Adults

Mei-Yi Wong[1], Chen Kang Lee[2], Paul E. Croarkin[3], and Poh Foong Lee[1(✉)]

[1] Lee Kong Chian Faculty of Engineering and Science, Universiti Tunku Abdul Rahman,
Kuala Lumpur, Malaysia
leepf@utar.edu.my

[2] Department of Information Systems, Faculty of Information and Communication Technology,
Universiti Tunku Abdul Rahman, Kampar Perak, Malaysia

[3] Department of Psychiatry and Psychology, Mayo Clinic, Rochester, MN, USA

Abstract. Depression is a common, but serious medical illness. Several influential cognitive theories propose that the maintenance of depressive symptoms is associated with negative cognitive biases. This study aims to evaluate the effectiveness of using a dot-probe task to detect negative attention bias in young adults and to study the effectiveness in using emoji images versus real face images in a dot-probe task. A total of 50 young adults (aged 18 to 29) were recruited and completed a visual dot-probe task under two conditions, once with face-type stimuli and then with emoji-type stimuli. Participants exhibiting depressive symptoms showed a greater attention bias towards faces with sad expressions compared to non-depressed participants. However, no evidence was found for differences in attention biases towards happy expressions, as well as toward emoji images representing happy and sad expressions. The average reaction time was faster for emoji-type trials compared to face-type trials. Results support the use of happy and sad expressions in a dot-probe task to detect attention bias related to depressive symptoms in young adults. Despite finding a lack of differences in general attention bias towards emoji-type images, further analysis is required to make a reliable verdict on the efficacy of using emoji images in a dot probe task.

Keywords: Dot-probe task · Depression · Young adults · Attention bias

1 Introduction

Depression is a prevalent and serious disorder with impairing symptoms such as fatigue, sleep disturbances, anger management issues, feelings of hopelessness and guilt, and thoughts of death and suicide [1]. Cognitive theories of depression have postulated that the development, maintenance and recurrence of depressive episodes are linked with negative cognitive biases [2–5]. Depression has been associated with the tendency to attend to negative words over positive or neutral words [6] as well as negative faces over positive or neutral faces [7, 8]. Depressed subjects have also been shown to have a reduced positive bias, which is present in non-depressed individuals [9]. Accordingly,

© Springer Nature Switzerland AG 2021
F. Ibrahim et al. (Eds.): ICIBEL 2019, IFMBE Proceedings 81, pp. 150–157, 2021.
https://doi.org/10.1007/978-3-030-65092-6_18

if attention bias is associated with the etiology of depressive symptoms, measuring the attention bias would aid in the detection of the disorder.

A dot-probe paradigm is the classic task used to measure attention bias, although modified versions exist for training purposes or to accommodate eye-tracking measurements. In a dot-probe task, a positive and negative stimulus appear on a computer screen simultaneously in two separate spatial locations. The stimuli are then vanished, and a dot probe appears in one of the locations where the stimuli was previously displayed. The subject's response time is recorded and a faster response to the probe when it appears in the previous location of a threatening stimulus is interpreted as a vigilance for threat, indicating attentional bias [10]. Current research on cognitive bias is focused on examining the role of attention bias in depression and developing effective experimental procedures for treatment. The development of more effective paradigms in the measurement of attention bias will contribute towards a useful clinical tool for depression, with added benefits of reduced cost.

This study aims to evaluate the dot-probe paradigm as a method of identifying symptoms of depression through detection of negative attention bias. Pictures of faces and emoji are used as the stimuli in the task. Dot-probe tasks used in past studies on attention bias in depression mainly utilize face pairs or word pairs. Recently, a diverse range of non-disorder specific images have been found to have an effect on cognitive biases related to emotional disorders [11]. Thus, this study will also investigate the effect of using emoji image pairs in a dot-probe task compared to the standard face image pairs.

2 Methods

2.1 Participants

A total of 50 participants were recruited for the study from university undergraduate and postgraduate students, aged between 18 to 29 years (mean = 21.80, SD = 2.44). Selective and convenience sampling methods were used to recruit participants mainly through social media network or by word of mouth. There were 28 participants in the depressive group and 22 participants in the control group. The exclusion criteria for the study were individuals with history of substance abuse, are currently on psychotropic medications or psychological therapy, or suffering symptoms of schizophrenia or neurological disorders.

2.2 Measures and Instruments

Questionnaires
Participants' depressive scores were assessed using the Depression and Anxiety Stress Scales (DASS-21). The DASS-21 is a shorter, 21-item version of the DASS and measures the magnitude of depression, anxiety and stress states [12]. The reliability (Cronbach's alpha) score for the DASS-21 Depression scale has been shown to be good, at 0.88 [13, 14]. Participants also completed the mood and anxiety modules from the Patient Health Questionnaire (PHQ-9 and GAD-7) (Spitzer, Williams and Kroenke) and the Oxford Happiness questionnaire [16]. The PHQ-9 scores 9 depression-related criteria from the

Patient Health Questionnaire, the GAD-7 scores 7 common anxiety symptoms and the Oxford Happiness questionnaire is a 29-item scale for assessing personal happiness.

Dot-probe Task

The dot-probe task in this experiment employed two types of stimuli, images of facial expressions and images of emoji. The faces stimuli consist of 16 sets of images selected from the NimStim Face Stimulus Set [17]. The chosen images were of closed-mouth expressions of 16 actors (9 female, 7 male) portraying Happy, Neutral and Sad expressions. The emoji images were created by JoyPixels and used under license [18]. Five emojis containing either the words "smiling" or "grinning" in their descriptions were chosen to depict happy emotions, while five emojis containing either the words "frowning", "disappointed" or "crying" in their descriptions were chosen to depict sad emotions. A neutral emoji was used to depict the neutral expression. All images were presented in greyscale.

All face image pairs consist of an emotional expression (either happy or sad) paired with the neutral expression of the same actor. Happy expressions are never paired with sad expressions. Therefore, the 32 face image pairs are presented about twice in every block for a total of 60 trials. The emoji image pairs also comprise of an emotional expression paired with the neutral expression. The 10 emoji image pairs are presented 6 times per block for a total of 60 trials. The order in which the image pairs appear in each block is fully randomized for every trial block.

2.3 Procedure

Participants were briefed on the study and given instructions for the task, after which written informed consent was obtained from them. Before starting with the dot-probe task, demographic information was collected from the participants. After that, participants completed the DASS-21, PHQ-9, GAD-7 and Oxford Happiness Questionnaire.

At the beginning of the dot-probe task, 12 practice trials were provided to enable the participants to familiarize themselves with the task. The actual experimental dot probe task consisted of 240 experimental trials divided into four blocks, each block separated by short breaks. Face pairs were presented as stimuli during the first two blocks of trials while emoji pairs were presented during the second two blocks of trials. Each trial began with a blank screen for 500 ms, after which a fixation dot was presented in the centre of the computer screen for 500 ms. A pair of faces were presented in a top-bottom alignment for 1000 ms. Once the face pair disappeared, a probe appeared with equal probability either in the top position or the bottom position. The probe had an equal probability of being the letter "Q" or the letter "O". The participant was required to press the "Q" key on the keyboard if a "Q" probe had appeared or press the "O" key if an "O" had appeared. The probe remained on the screen until the participant pressed one of the corresponding keys or timeout of the trial at occurred 3000 ms.

The response time and accuracy of the participant in each trial was recorded. The emotional expression had an equal probability of appearing either in the top position or the bottom position. The task was conducted on each participant individually on a computer in a laboratory testing room. The experiment sessions lasted between 50 min to 1 h each. Participants were provided details on the purpose of the study at the end of the sessions.

2.4 Data Analysis

Bias Index Calculation

The dot probe task was implemented using OpenSesame [19]. During the task, the program recorded the reaction times for each trial. The reaction times were used to calculate an attention bias score using the following equation [6]:

$$Bias\,score = \frac{1}{2}[(UT * LP + LT * UP) - (UT * UP + LT * LP)] \qquad (1)$$

where the term UT * LP corresponds to the reaction time of the subject when the probe is in the lower position (LP) and the threat, which is an emotional face in the case of this study, is in the upper position (UT). Therefore, (UT * LP + LT * UP) gives the reaction times for the incongruent trials where the probe appears in the opposite location from the emotional face, while (UT * UP + LT * LP) gives the reaction times for the congruent trials where the probe appears in the location of the emotion face. By subtracting the congruent trial reaction times from the incongruent trial reaction times, the mean speeding of response to threat can be calculated [20]. The bias score reflects the Threat Position x Probe Position interaction, with positive values indicating an attention bias towards threat (vigilance) and negative values indication a bias away from threat (avoidance).

In calculating the attention bias scores, only data from the dot-bottom trials were used. It was previously found that analyzing dot-bottom trials alone increased the reliability of the bias index even though the number of trials considered were halved [21]. The eye gaze of participants may be naturally drawn to the top half of the screen, possibly contributing to a bias which is unrelated to the disorder.

Statistics

Analysis of the data was carried out using the statistical package SPSS for Windows version 21 [22]. Shapiro-Wilk tests were used to verify the deviation from normal distribution for each bias index. T-Tests for independent samples were used to compare the depressive and non-depressive participants with respect to their attention bias indexes.

3 Results

3.1 Data Screening

All error trials were excluded from analyses. The number of errors made by participants ranged from 0 to 17 ($M = 5.04$, $SD = 4.11$). Errors occurred on 2.10% of all trials. Analyses were performed on the remaining data.

3.2 Demographics

Of the total sample of 50 participants, 23 were female and 27 were male. To check if there was a difference in proportion of females and males who were depressive or non-depressive, a 2 × 2 Chi-square test was conducted. The test revealed no significant association between gender of the participant and their condition, X2 (1, N = 50) = 0.41, p = .52. Therefore, any potential effects associated with gender should have been adjusted across both groups.

3.3 Attention Bias Indexes

Table 1 shows the mean reaction times and attention bias indexes of all participants for both types of stimuli. Shapiro-Wilk tests show that the attention bias indexes with face images as the stimuli follow a normal distribution, while the attention bias indexes for the dot probe task with emoji images deviate from a normal distribution.

Table 1. Bias indexes for non-depressive and depressive subjects.

Stimulus type	Bias index	Non-depressive subjects		Depressive subjects	
		Mean	SD	Mean	SD
Face trials	Happy	13.21	42.29	0.34	47.15
	Sad	− 3.76	44.31	12.26	41.86
Emoji trials	Happy	2.63	61.91	− 4.29	56.92
	Sad	− 18.97	75.37	− 4.16	37.27

For the dot-probe task using face images as the stimuli, independent t-tests were performed on the bias indexes between the depressed and non-depressed groups. The t-test indicated that the negative bias scores for the non-depressed group (−7.48) was statistically significantly lower compared to the depressed group (16.76), t(46) = −2.186, p = .034. On the other hand, results showed that there was no statistically significant difference in positive bias scores between the two groups.

Table 2. Reaction times for depressive and non-depressive subjects.

Stimulus type	Bias index	All subjects		Non-depressive subjects		Depressive subjects	
		Mean	SD	Mean	SD	Mean	SD
Face trials	Happy	621.41	127.59	620.57	133.67	622.07	125.09
	Sad	602.02	110.34	601.85	119.22	602.15	105.07
Emoji trials	Happy	611.71	116.65	611.21	124.75	612.11	112.21
	Sad	621.41	127.59	620.57	133.67	622.07	125.09

Since the values of the bias indexes for the dot-probe task using emoji images do not follow a normal distribution, the Mann-Whitney U test was used here. The results show that there was no statistically significant difference in negative or positive bias scores between the depressed and non-depressed groups.

3.4 Reaction Times

Table 2 shows the reaction times for all participants, by trial type. A Wilcoxon Signed Ranks test was used to examine if there were any differences in reaction times of participants under the face-type trials and the emoji-type trials conditions.

4 Discussion

The aims of this study were evaluate the effectiveness of using a dot-probe task to detect negative attention bias in young adults and to investigate the effect of using emoji images in a dot-probe task compared to standard face images. This study found that the presence of depressive symptoms affects the detection of sad facial expressions in images of human faces. This is in line with previous studies on depression and bias towards sad expressions [7, 23, 24]. Conversely, there was lack of difference found in attention biases towards happy expressions, in contrast to previous studies which have found evidence of a reduced or absent positive bias in depressed individuals [11, 25]. Given the relatively long presentation duration of the stimuli images in this study, the reaction times recorded included the effects of attention disengagement, as participants would have had enough time to make saccades between the two images displayed. It is possible that a difference in vigilance towards positive faces exists between the two groups, hence the congruent and incongruent indexes should be considered in further analyses.

The results did not show a general attention bias effect for sad or happy expressions in images of emoji. In addition to considering the effects of attention vigilance versus attention disengagement as detailed above, emoji images are comparatively different from images of facial expressions which may cause emojis to be less disorder-specific. It was found that the average reaction time of participants for emoji-type trials was faster than for the face-type trials. This may be an indication that participants had less trouble disengaging their attention from the images.

There are several limitations in the present study that should be noted. A large number of trials were used, which might have induced fatigue in the participants. In order to reduce this effect, the study design included several breaks in between the blocks of trials. Although blocking of trials is a common method used in dot-probe studies [26, 27], there is evidence that that the results may be affected, in terms of semantic relatedness [28]. Furthermore, the trial blocks were presented in such a way that participants completed the dot-probe task with face images as stimuli before completing the task with emoji images as stimuli. There may be a temporal aspect to attention bias which affected the performance of participants across the dot-probe task. Lastly, our sample was nonclinical, therefore the severity of depressive symptoms may not correspond to that of a clinical sample.

Future analyses of the data should take into account vigilance/avoidance effects and separate them from disengagement effects. Additionally, in the trial block order could be randomized for each participant in future studies to address the possible effects of fatigue on the performance of participants on the emoji dot-probe task.

5   Conclusion

In conclusion, the present study provides further evidence that individuals exhibiting depressive symptoms show an attention bias towards negatively-valenced emotional faces. The results support the use of happy and sad facial expressions in the dot-probe task for detecting negative attention bias in young adults. Although a difference in general attention bias was not found towards emoji-type images, more analyses is required to further investigate the vigilance and disengagement components of attention under this condition.

References

1. National Institute of Mental Health: Depression, National Institute of Mental Health, https://www.nimh.nih.gov/health/topics/depression/index.shtml, last accessed 2018/01/17
2. Beck, A.T.: Cognitive therapy and the emotional disorders. International Universities Press, Oxford (1976)
3. Beck, A.T.: The Evolution of the Cognitive Model of Depression and Its Neurobiological Correlates. Am. J. Psychiatry 165(8), 969–977 (2008)
4. Mathews, A., MacLeod, C.: Cognitive Vulnerability to Emotional Disorders. Ann. Rev. Clin. Psychol. 1(1), 167–195 (2005)
5. Clark, D.A., Beck, A.T., Alford, B.A.: Scientific Foundations of Cognitive Theory and Therapy of Depression. and Alford. Wiley, New York (1999)
6. Bradley, B.P., Mogg, K., Lee, S.C.: Attentional biases for negative information in induced and naturally occurring dysphoria. Behav. Res. Ther. 35(10), 911–927 (1997)
7. Joormann, J., Gotlib, I.H.: Selective attention to emotional faces following recovery from depression. J. Abnorm. Psychol. 116(1), 80–85 (2007)
8. Leyman, L., De Raedt, R., Schacht, R., Koster, E.H.W.: Attentional biases for angry faces in unipolar depression. Psychol. Med. 37(03), 393 (2007)
9. Duque, A., Vázquez, C.: Double attention bias for positive and negative emotional faces in clinical depression: Evidence from an eye-tracking study. J. Behav. Ther. Exp. Psychiatry. Pergamon 46, 107–114 (2015)
10. Hakamata, Y., Lissek, S., Bar-Haim, Y., Britton, J.C., Fox, N.A., Leibenluft, E., Ernst, M., Pine, D.S.: Attention bias modification treatment: a meta-analysis toward the establishment of novel treatment for anxiety. Biol. Psychiatry. NIH Public Access 68(11), 982–990 (2010)
11. Becker, E.S., Ferentzi, H., Ferrari, G., Möbius, M., Brugman, S., Custers, J., Geurtzen, N., Wouters, J., Rinck, M.: Always approach the bright side of life: a general positivity training reduces stress reactions in vulnerable individuals. Cogn. Ther. Res. 40(1), 57–71 (2016)
12. Parkitny, L., McAuley, J.: The depression anxiety stress scale (DASS). Journal of Physiotherapy 56(3), 204 (2010)
13. Henry, J.D., Crawford, J.R.: The short-form version of the Depression Anxiety Stress Scales (DASS-21): Construct validity and normative data in a large non-clinical sample. British J. Clin. Psychology 44(2), 227–239 (2005)

14. Sinclair, S.J., Siefert, C.J., Slavin-Mulford, J.M., Stein, M.B., Renna, M., Blais, M.A.: Psychometric evaluation and normative data for the depression, anxiety, and stress scales-21 (DASS-21) in a nonclinical sample of U.S. adults. Eval. Health Prof. **35**(3), 259–279 (2012)
15. Spitzer, R.L., Williams, J.B.W., Kroenke, K.: Instructions for Patient Health Questionnaire (PHQ) and GAD-7 Measures Accessed 14 Dec 2018
16. Hills, P., Argyle, M.: The oxford happiness questionnaire: a compact scale for the measurement of psychological well-being. Pers. Individ. Differ. Pergamon **33**(7), 1073–1082 (2002)
17. Tottenham, N., Tanaka, J.W., Leon, A.C., McCarry, T., Nurse, M., Hare, T.A., Marcus, D.J., Westerlund, A., Casey, B., Nelson, C.: The NimStim set of facial expressions: Judgments from untrained research participants. Psychiatry Res. **168**(3), 242–249 (2009)
18. JoyPixels 2017 Emoji Set, https://www.joypixels.com/emoji/v3 Accessed 27 Sep 2019
19. Mathôt, S., Schreij, D., Theeuwes, J., Theeuwes, J.: OpenSesame: an open-source, graphical experiment builder for the social sciences. Behav. Res. Methods. Springer-Verlag **44**(2), 314–324 (2012)
20. Mogg, K., Mathews, A., Eysenck, M.: Attentional bias to threat in clinical anxiety states. Cogn. Emot. **6**(2), 149–159 (1992)
21. Price, R.B., Kuckertz, J.M., Siegle, G.J., Ladouceur, C.D., Silk, J.S., Ryan, N.D., Dahl, R.E., Amir, N.: Empirical recommendations for improving the stability of the dot-probe task in clinical research. Psychol. Assess. NIH Publ. Access **27**(2), 365–376 (2015)
22. IBM Corp.: IBM SPSS Statistics for Windows. Armonk, NY: IBM Corp (2012)
23. Gotlib, I.H., Krasnoperova, E., Yue, D.N., Joormann, J.: Attentional biases for negative interpersonal stimuli in clinical depression. J. Abnorm. Psychol. **113**(1), 127–135 (2004)
24. Wells, T.T., Beevers, C.G.: Biased attention and dysphoria: Manipulating selective attention reduces subsequent depressive symptoms. Cogn. Emot. **24**(4), 719–728 (2010)
25. Baert, S., De Raedt, R., Schacht, R., Koster, E.H.W.: Attentional bias training in depression: Therapeutic effects depend on depression severity. J. Behav. Ther. Exp. Psychiatry **41**(3), 265–274 (1976)
26. Donaldson, C., Lam, D., Mathews, A.: Rumination and attention in major depression. Behav. Res. Ther. **45**(11), 2664–2678 (2007)
27. Schmidt, N.B., Richey, J.A., Buckner, J.D., Timpano, K.R.: Attention Training for Generalized Social Anxiety Disorder. J. Abnorm. Psychol. **118**(1), 5 (2009)
28. Keogh, E., Cheng, F., Wang, S.: Exploring attentional biases towards facial expressions of pain in men and women. Eur. J. Pain **22**(9), 1617–1627 (2018)

Optimal Driving Current for Improved Noninvasive Near Infrared Glucose Meter

Mohammed Omar, Mohd Yazed Ahmad$^{(\boxtimes)}$, and Wan Safwani Wan Kamarul Zaman

University of Malaya, 59200 Kuala Lumpur, Malaysia
myaz@um.edu.my

Abstract. Diabetes is one of common diseases nowadays that associated with inability of human body to control level of glucose in the body. The danger of the diabetes can be minimized by continuously monitor the glucose level of the patient. There are several methods to measure the glucose level in the blood either invasive, minimally invasive or non-invasive method. In this paper, we conducted an experiment using non-invasive near infrared approach to investigate the relationship between the level of the glucose and the corresponding sensing parameters. We used infrared LED as emitter and receiver. They are positioned opposite to each other with the sample in between. The LED transmitter driving current was varied from 40 mA up to 80 mA. There were 14 different level of glucose concentration were used as samples. We performed analysis on the collected received signals at the receiver when glucose level and LED driving current were varied. The results revealed that there is a linear relationship between the current applied to the LED and the received signal also known as sensing voltage. Different values of current applied to the transmitting infrared LED gave different levels of accuracy of glucose prediction. The optimal driving current was found at 60 mA, which provides the best accuracy as compared to 40 mA and 80 mA. In other words, 60 mA current has highest correlation factor and lowest error percentage.

Keywords: Infrared LED · Blood glucose measurement · Optimal infrared driving current

1 Introduction

Diabetes is one of the common and crucial disease caused by the deficiency of the insulin level in the blood. Diabetes might lead to other health issues such as heart attack, heart failure, and kidney failure. Statistics shows that there are 285 million cases of diabetes, and according to World Health Organization (WHO), the number will increase to 366 million by 2030. Therefore, it is important to keep monitoring the glucose level in the blood in order to predict any dramatic changes of the glucose – hyperglycemia or hypoxia – and to prevent it before it happens. There are three main ways to measure the glucose concentration in the blood; invasive, minimally invasive and non-invasive methods.

Invasive method is the most common approach in the hospitals nowadays. Invasive measurement involves pricking a finger to get a drop of blood, and then transfer it to the blood test strip [1]. This method is painful and the wound recovery process for the

© Springer Nature Switzerland AG 2021
F. Ibrahim et al. (Eds.): ICIBEL 2019, IFMBE Proceedings 81, pp. 158–164, 2021.
https://doi.org/10.1007/978-3-030-65092-6_19

diabetic people does not happen fast which may cause an infection [2, 3]. Also, the test strip is disposable which may increase the cost. Minimally invasive approaches is another way that cause less pain in comparison to the invasive method. Many methods have been suggested for the minimal invasive such as iontophoresis, microdialysis and biosensor implementation [3–7].

Non-invasive method is the most convenient way because it is painless and it does not required test strips [8]. Recently, more non-invasive ways were introduced such as Near Infrared (NIR), Mid Infrared Spectroscope (Mid-IR) [9], and Raman spectroscope [10]. NIR is a light concept which depends on emitting a beam of light that has certain wavelength, typically in the range of 750–2500 nm [11]. The body absorbs and scatter the light due to the interaction with the chemical composition of the tissue. The NIR detect the measurement within depth range of 1–100 mm deep [12].

The reduction of the light intensity as it travels through the tissue is explained by the light transparent theory. According to the equation, $I = Io \, ee^{-\mu eff d}$, where I is reflected light, Io is incident light, μeff is the effective light reduction, and d is the optical path length [13]. Then, the light will be reflected from the tissue and received by a photodiode that converts light to voltage. The difference in glucose concentration is described by the variation of the voltage obtained by the photodiode. In other words, the glucose will block the light that passed through the tissue based on glucose concentration [14]. A previous study compared the NIR method with Raman spectroscopy and concluded that NIR is more appropriate and can generate accurate measurements. The lack of accuracy of Raman spectroscopy method was attributed to the accumulation of noise that interfere during the measurement [15, 16].

According to [17], he carried an experiment by passing a light through one side of the finger and the reflected light from the other side of the finger was considered to describe the amount of light in the blood glucose.

In a previous study [18], a comparison between two different wavelength ranges (750–2500 nm and 1000–2500 nm) was performed. The study concluded that 750–2500 is the infrared band, and any wavelength under 1000 nm gives inaccurate result [19]. Another study suggested a wavelength between 1100 nm and 2450 nm [20].

Experiments were conducted to measure the glucose concentration as voltage function and a linear relation between the sensing voltage and the glucose concentration was reported [21–24]. However, the influence of the current driving to the LED on the performance of the glucometer is not being fully investigated. Therefore, in this paper, we investigated the relationship between the current value and the accuracy of blood glucose measurement by using the NIR method. The voltage was fixed and the current was changed to 40 mA, 60 mA and 80 mA. The main objective of this was to find the best fitting current value that gives more accurate prediction of the glucose concentration.

2 Materials and Methodology

Two NIR LEDs were used in the experiment: emitter and receiver. The emitter is an infrared LED (LED1550E) that has a wavelength range of 1400–1650 nm. The receiver is a photodiode (FGA10) that has a wavelength range of 900–1700 nm and it is capable of converting light to voltage. The two LEDs were positioned directly opposite to each other. The emitter was connected to the power supply. The voltage was fixed at1.5 V, and three different current values were applied: 40 mA, 60 mA and 80 mA. According to the data sheet of the LED1550E, the maximum current for the LED is 100 mA.

Glucose concentrations were prepared using the dilution serial [serial]. 14 solutions were prepared: [40,60,80,100,120,140,160,180,200,220,240,260,280,300] mg/dL and the solutions were contained in a test tube. First measurement was collected when the current is 40 mA, then 60 and the last measurement was at 80 mA. The temperature of the sample was fixed to room temperature. The voltage reading was captured using a Multimeter that connected to the photodiode.

Data analysis tools were used such as linear regression, mean square error, correlation error percentage to study the relationship between the current value and the accuracy or the prediction of the glucose concentration.

3   Result and Discussion

Table 1 indicates a linear relationship between the glucose concentration and the output voltage; the sensing voltage increases indirect proportion with the glucose level – this is supported by previous research studied [21–24]. Also, the constant raise of the voltage when we increase the current is explained by the Ohm's.

Table 1. Shows the output voltage with different driving current

Mg/dl	Current 40 mA	Current 60 mA	Current 80 mA
40	137.3	147.7	153.1
60	137.6	147.9	153.5
80	139	148.4	152.8
100	141.6	149	153
120	142.8	149.4	154
140	142.4	149.6	154.1
160	143.3	149.8	154.2
180	144.4	150	154.3
200	145.2	151.3	154.7
220	145.4	151.4	155
240	145.2	151.9	155.2
260	145.1	152.3	155.3
280	144.8	152.8	155.7
300	145.7	153.4	156.7

Table 2 shows the correlation, mean square error, linear equation and the error percentage of each experiment. According to the Fig. 4, we can notice that MSE, correlation,

and raises at 40 mA and then reach the peak at 60 mA and drop back again at 80 mA. Since correlation and MSE indicates a better relationship when they are bigger, so 60 mA gives the most significant linear relationship. According to the datasheet of the LED1550E, the maximum current that is applicable for the LED is 100 mA. According to [25], the higher the current value applied to the light emitting diode the less efficiency of the LED decreases. Moreover, looking at Table 2, 60 mA has a very small percentage error compared to 80 mA and 40 mA. Looking at the overall analysis, we can conclude that driving current at 60 mA provides the best fitting and optimal compared to 40 mA and 80 mA (Figs. 1, 2 and 3).

Table 2. shows the correlation, MSE, erorr percentage and the linear equation of each sample

	40 mA	60 mA	80 mA
Correlation factor	92%	99%	96%
Linear equation	Y = 25.3 x −3439.1	Y = 45.103 x −6611.2	Y = 83.193x −12686
Means square error	86%	98%	93%
Error percentage	− 2.6%	− 0.04%	3.3%

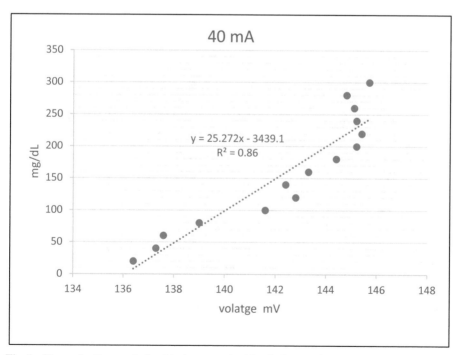

Fig. 1. Shows the linear relationship between the blood glcucose level and the output voltage with driving current of 40 mA

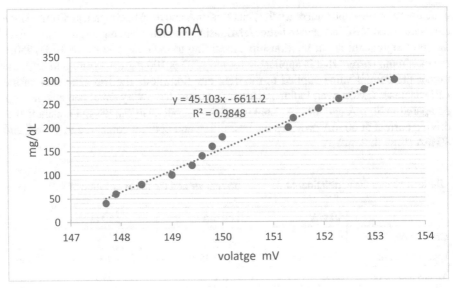

Fig. 2. Shows the linear relationship between the blood glcucose level and the output voltage with driving current of 60 mA

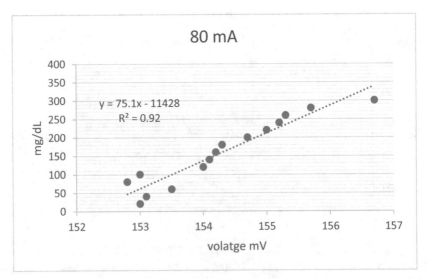

Fig. 3. Shows the linear relationship between the blood glcucose level and the output voltage with driving current of 80 mA

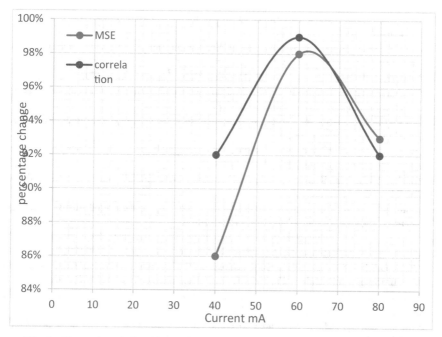

Fig. 4. Shows the relationship between the current values with Correlation and MSE

4   Conclusion

Constant monitoring of the blood glucose is important to avoid the complications of the diabetes. Plenty ways to do that such as the invasive and non-invasive. So far, the noninvasive is the best approach. In this experiment, we conducted a study in the non-invasive approaches using the NIR, we applied different current values to the emitter to study the significant of the current values to the blood glucose prediction. We found out that the higher accuracy of the blood glucose concentration can be obtained by applying 60 mA current to the emitter. Future work can be carried to investigate the relationship between the glucose temperature – or patient temperature – and the glucose measurement.

References

1. Phillips, R. et al.: No-wipe whole blood glucose test strip. 1995, Google Patents
2. Brem, H., Tomic-Canic, M.: Cellular and molecular basis of wound healing in diabetes. Journal of clinical investigation **117**(5), 1219–1222 (2007)
3. Hopkins, G.W., Mauze, G.R.: In-vivo NIR diffuse-reflectance tissue spectroscopy of human subjects. in Optical Tomography and Spectroscopy of Tissue III. 1999. International Society for Optics and Photonics
4. Leboulanger, B., Guy, R.H., Delgado-Charro, M.B.: Reverse iontophoresis for non-invasive transdermal monitoring. Physiol. Meas. **25**(3), R35 (2004)

5. Rhee, S.Y., et al.: Clinical experience of an iontophoresis based glucose measuring system. **22**(1), 70–73 (2007)
6. Klonoff, D.C.: Microdialysis of interstitial fluid for continuous glucose measurement. 2003, Mary Ann Liebert, Inc
7. Bolincier, J., Ungerstedt, U., Arner, P.J.D.: Microdialysis measurement of the absolute glucose concentration in subcutaneous adipose tissue allowing glucose monitoring in diabetic patients. Diabetologia **35**(12), 1177–1180 (1992)
8. do Amaral, C.E., Wolf, B.: Current development in non-invasive glucose monitoring. Med. Eng. Phys. **30**(5), 541–549 (2008)
9. Liakat, S., et al.: Noninvasive in vivo glucose sensing on human subjects using mid-infrared light. Biomed. Opt. Express **5**(7), 2397–2404 (2014)
10. Enejder, A.M., et al.: Raman spectroscopy for noninvasive glucose measurements. J. Biomed. Opt. **10**(3), 031114 (2005)
11. Malin, S.F., et al.: Noninvasive prediction of glucose by near-infrared diffuse reflectance spectroscopy. Clin. Chem. **45**(9), 1651–1658 (1999)
12. Tura, A., et al.: Non-invasive glucose monitoring: assessment of technologies and devices according to quantitative criteria. Diabetes Res. Clin. Pract. **77**(1), 16–40 (2007)
13. Khalil, O.S.: Non-invasive glucose measurement technologies: an update from 1999 to the dawn of the new millennium. Diabetes Tech. Therapeutics **6**(5), 660–697 (2004)
14. Amir, O., et al.: Continuous noninvasive glucose monitoring technology based on "occlusion spectroscopy". SAGE Publications (2007)
15. Shin, K., Chung, H.J.A.: Wide area coverage raman spectroscopy for reliable quantitative analysis and its applications. Analyst **138**(12), 3335–3346 (2013)
16. Rossi, E.E., et al.: Differential diagnosis between experimental endophthalmitis and uveitis in vitreous with Raman spectroscopy and principal components analysis. J. Photochem. Photobiol. B Biol. **107**, 73–78 (2012)
17. Shinde, A.A., Prasad, R.K.: Non invasive blood glucose measurement using NIR technique based on occlusion spectroscopy. Int. J. Eng. Sci. Tech. (IJEST) **3**(12), 8325–8333 (2011)
18. Waynant, R.W., Chenault, V.M.: Overview of non-invasive fluid glucose measurement using optical techniques to maintain glucose control in diabetes mellitus. IEEE LEOS Newsl. **12**(2), 3–6 (1998)
19. Kajiwara, K., et al.: Noninvasive measurement of blood glucose concentrations by analysing fourier transform infra-red absorbance spectra through oral mucosa. Med. Biol. Eng. Comput. **31**(1), S17–S22 (1993)
20. Jeon, K.J., et al.: Comparison between transmittance and reflectance measurements in glucose determination using near infrared spectroscopy. J. Biom. Opt. **11**(1), 014022 (2006)
21. Asekar, M.S.: Development of Portable Non-Invasive Blood Glucose Measuring Device Using NIR Spectroscopy. In: 2018 Second International Conference on Intelligent Computing and Control Systems (ICICCS), IEEE (2018)
22. Buda, R.A., Addi, M.M.: A portable non-invasive blood glucose monitoring device. In: 2014 IEEE Conference on Biomedical Engineering and Sciences (IECBES), IEEE (2014)
23. Daarani, P., Kavithamani, A.: Blood glucose level monitoring by noninvasive method using near infrared sensor. J. Latest Trends Eng. Technol. 141–147 (2017). https://doi.org/10.21172/1.IRES.19
24. Rahmat, M.A. et al.: GluQo: IoT-based non-invasive blood glucose monitoring **9**(3–9), 71-75 (2017)
25. Malyutenko, V., et al.: Current crowding in InAsSb light-emitting diodes. Appl. Phys. Lett. **79**(25), 4228–4230 (2001)

Author Index

© Springer Nature Switzerland AG 2021
F. Ibrahim et al. (Eds.): ICIBEL 2019, IFMBE Proceedings 81, pp. 165–166, 2021.
https://doi.org/10.1007/978-3-030-65092-6

Printed in the United States
By Bookmasters